'An important, timely and powerful
be "normal" and how to release ou
that word.' – **Fran Bushe**, author of

'A beautiful yet brutally honest account of a woman's journey to
accepting herself. Raw, funny, candid – you'll be whisked through the
pages with Ally's voice in your head as she navigates the shock of her
diagnosis as a teenager, shame as she grapples with it, self-destruction
as a coping mechanism but ultimately acceptance and self-discovery.
This is a book for all women. It covers so many key topics about our
roles in society, relationships, intimacy and so much more. I read it in
one go!' – **Isla Traquair**, award-winning journalist and broadcaster

'A breathtakingly honest, raw and surprisingly funny memoir about
what it means for society to question your identity.' – **Amy Molloy**,
journalist and author of *Wife, Interrupted*

'Everyone has a vagina story, whether we have a vagina or not. The
word is shrouded in stigma – hidden and censored just like our stories,
untold and buried in shame. The power in this narrative untangles
so many layers of society, from poor sex education to defining
womanhood and unlearning our pre-defined roles. Ally's story, a story
I share as another womb-less, vagina-less woman, touches so many
hearts stuck in this binary world; from sex, gender and bodies, all the
things that shouldn't have a rule book. It amplifies the message that
we are no less. It teaches us that there's no one way to be a girl, or a
woman, or a person – we aren't in a contract with society. It's a vagina
story that queefs away the patriarchal definition of "woman" but that
gives a big labia-hug to trauma, self-esteem and mental health.'
– **Ellamae Fullalove**, creator of Va Va Womb, and sex and body
positivity social media influencer

First published in 2024 by Ally Hensley,
in partnership with Whitefox Publishing

www.wearewhitefox.com

Copyright © Ally Hensley, 2024

ISBN 978-1-916797-76-5
Also available as an eBook
ISBN 978-1-916797-77-2

Edited by Amy Molloy
Copy-edited by Gina Rathbone
Designed and typeset by Karen Lilje
Cover design by Emma Ewbank
Project management by Whitefox

VAGINA UNCENSORED

A Memoir of Missing Parts

ALLY HENSLEY

To my mummie,
Me: Thank you for listening.
You: Always.
I love you.

To my daddy, my 'partner in crime and DIY',
I love you.

To the MRKH community, we are all so brave,
I love you.

And Esme, I'm not quite sure where you are, but thank
you for choosing me.
One day, I'd love for us to finally meet.

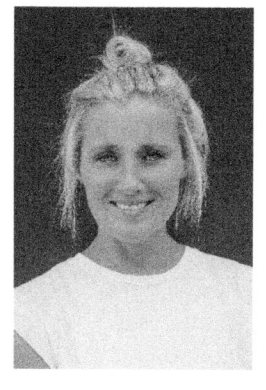

Ally Hensley is an author, speaker, stigma shaker and global ambassador for women's health and happiness. Ally has written for leading publications on mental health, infertility and body positivity, and has become a regular media contributor on her experience of being born with MRKH, a medical condition resulting in the absence of a womb and vagina.

In 2020, Ally co-produced the first short film about MRKH, alongside a leading digital storytelling brand, featuring women from across the globe who bravely shared experiences with MRKH. This film premiered at the World Congress for Paediatric and Adolescent Gynaecology in 2019, exposing the experiences of seven women across the globe as they told their unique and complex stories of their MRKH diagnosis.

As an international spokesperson for MRKH on how to redefine womanhood on her own terms, Ally advocates to raise support and awareness of this life-altering diagnosis. She founded Australia's first MRKH organisation, MRKH Australia, in 2013, co-founded Global MRKH in 2016 and is a board member of the UK's flagship charity, MRKH Connect.

Her podcast *Stigma Shakers* recently launched, and just two seasons in, this stigma-focused show has been featured by the BBC, among many other national publications, and has reached over 150k views. Now, *Stigma Shakers* is recognised as not just a taboo-tackling platform, but a social movement, in questioning: 'Is the only thing normal in this world difference?'

Ally works to reduce the stigma surrounding sexual (mental) health and prompts conversations that matter. She defines herself as a realistic but scrappy dreamer – where fact is essential, and originality is to be absolutely embraced.

Contents

SOUNDTRACK

Rarely will you see me without a pair of earphones, listening to music, be it strolling down the street, twitching in a doctor's waiting room or dragging my heels to buy a pint of milk. On the flip side, I've pressed 'play' on some of the most magical times of my life: getting a book deal, making love, mending hearts, and all the moments where my big feelings have surfaced.

I need music like I need therapy.

Because music, for me, is everything.

Aside from wanting to become a renowned courtroom lawyer, famous actress and *of course bestselling author* (you gotta manifest the shit out of life!), my other occupation of choice was to be a sound composer, who engineers the soundtracks for blockbuster movies.

When I decided to write this book, I knew music would be my emotive accomplice. With every chapter written, I selected a song that was not only fitting to my mood of the moment, but that was evocative of the year in which the chapter plays out.

If, like me, you are someone who needs music to be a backdrop to a difficult or hopeful day, I have created a soundtrack to this book for you.

In turn, this playlist has become the soundtrack to my life.

Simply search for Ally Hensley on Spotify and drop into the chapters with me. So, when you're ready, please press ... play.

Happy listening.

ACCESS THE PLAYLIST ON SPOTIFY
Open Spotify app, tap Search, use the camera icon to scan the
Spotify Code and the playlist will open automatically.

INTRODUCTION
Coldplay: 'Fix You'

CHAPTER 1
Alanis Morissette: 'You Learn'
Scala & Kolacny Brothers: 'With or Without You'

CHAPTER 2
Massive Attack: 'Teardrop'
Primal Scream: 'Come Together'

CHAPTER 3
Sarah Brightman: 'Deliver Me'
Ocean Colour Scene: 'Lining Your Pockets'

CHAPTER 4
Embrace: 'Come Back to What You Know'
Stephen Gately: 'I Believe'

CHAPTER 5
The Killers: 'Glamorous Indie Rock & Roll'
U2: 'Stuck in a Moment You Can't Get Out Of'

CHAPTER 6
The Darkness: 'Love Is Only a Feeling'
The Streets: 'Dry Your Eyes'

CHAPTER 7
The Chicks: 'Not Ready to Make Nice'
Blessid Union of Souls: 'I Believe'

Making my vagina

I will preface this chapter by saying you are going to read the word 'vagina' a lot throughout this book. Not because I am a sexologist, healthcare professional or sex worker, but because, for the last 26 years, this body part (or once, the lack thereof) has been at the centre of my identity struggle.

I am not trying to shock you or hook a headline. I am not trying to kick-start a global campaign about gender rights. I certainly am not wanting to offend you or trigger unhealed wounds. I am simply wanting, and ready, to tell my story so that someday, this word doesn't cause someone else the grief that it caused me.

It's crazy, really, that I would allow anatomy to redefine my life on a monthly, if not weekly, basis. But, to all intents and purposes, it did. In some ways, it still does. Because, without the word 'vagina', my life wouldn't have taken the twists and turns it has today; some good, some devastating and some incredibly liberating. Weird, right?

I was just a few months into my 'sweet sixteen' when I was told that I had been born without a womb, cervix and a vagina – a medical condition widely termed MRKH, or Müllerian agenesis (meaning 'absence of').

Interestingly, the term 'sweet sixteen' derives from a Latin American milestone, where families celebrate a girl transitioning from childhood into womanhood.

The pressure!

For me, sweet it was not.

At the peak of my adolescence, I was given clear evidence I was different – and different in a way that wasn't politically correct to talk about. While my girlfriends were whispering about getting their first periods, I was told I was never going to achieve this rite of passage. If I didn't take extreme steps, I could never have sex. My body would never be able to naturally carry a baby.

I was still a child, having to unlearn, unsee, unhear and unfeel everything that I had believed my future as a woman would look like. Every magazine article, Judy Blume book, film, TV show and overheard conversation from the women around me was to be utterly rocked and reduced to emotional rubble.

There I was, grieving my life as a woman, as a child.

This is the story of what happened next – a story about shame, self-identity, sexual exploration and what it really means to be a woman, when you don't tick all the boxes of what a woman is.

SAME SHAME, DIFFERENT DAY ...

I've been staring at this blank page for 42 years.

As a professional writer and the creator of a not-for-profit supporting women with MRKH, writing a book about my journey has been the obvious step for years – but it was not a path I was eager to take.

Every time I was asked, 'When are you going to write a book?' I would reply, 'When I am done with gathering content.' This was code for: I am still healing from my gaping wounds; I am still healing from broken hearts; I am still grieving what I thought my life would look like; and I am still grieving my lost womanhood.

When I said 'gathering content', what I meant was: I'm still trying to gather myself.

It has taken me a long time – a lifetime – to even begin to understand who I am, alongside the diagnosis that rocked my world. There have been spells when I've thought I'd never be ready to write 'the book' but then, somewhere during the pandemic and after my fortieth birthday, I got there.

Now, I am ready to share my story with you.

I am ready to completely untangle the trauma I experienced as a 16-year-old girl, the dark days, the really dark days, the moments where I finally made sense of my pain and how I became a person on a mission to answer one, unshakeable question: when will I feel like a woman?

I'm Ally Hensley; a daughter, sister, aunt, lover, professional writer, speaker, editor and reiki healer. There were only two – well, three – dream jobs I had as a teenager: a lawyer, an Oscar-winning actress and a writer. As a serial school dropout, I never did make law or theatre school. Instead, I chose to become a grafter. I became a dish pig (slang: kitchen hand), pub manager, IT support worker (don't even ask me how I landed that gig) and a fancily booted corporate ice-queen.

But words? Words I can do. Words I love.

Words have this magical way of travelling to the people who need them the most. Words can paint a picture that we cannot always vocalise. And the more honest these words are, the better our hearts will be. If only truth was as trendy as TikTok (that's a topic for a later chapter!).

So, here I am, sipping a coffee, on a Monday morning, listening to Coldplay and writing my debut memoir. It feels like I am meeting a long-lost relative, seeing a fantasy come to life or going on a first date with someone I've had a massive crush on for such a long time. It's so exciting, but equally terrifying.

The pressure to impress you may get in the way now and again. That's the people-pleaser in me. I am, however, proud of who I am today. Though it's not always been that way. In fact, for much of my life, I have lived in a body and head space that I wanted to evacuate regularly. I have lived in shame, secrecy, societal displacement and too much unhappiness.

Now, I am prepared to face fear, isolation, worthiness and my past head-on.

THE DAY MY VAGINA WENT VIRAL

You could say it was an extreme time of exposure therapy – sharing the most secret part of my story on the internet. In a later chapter, we'll talk about why, how and what led me to make an Instagram reel about how I made my own vagina – and how that reel became a viral sensation.

For now, the most important thing to know is: I know how it feels to carry guilt, shame and even hatred for yourself, for much of your life ... and then finally be seen. I understand, more than anyone, the complex relationship we can have with our body and ourselves, and the relief when you finally accept who you are.

As humans, we are never completely cured of our past, but we can make sense of it. We cannot live in the past, nor can we forget it. While I am not defined by my past, it has shaped the person I am today. If we are lucky enough, because healing isn't a given for everyone, we will get a chance to surrender to what has hurt us the most. We can break enough to understand the pain, but our hope can be big enough to remedy what broke us in the first place.

That's how I see my medical diagnosis.

4

In the next 17 chapters, you won't only hear my story, but you'll be nudged to really look at your own. What makes up the puzzle pieces of our identity; what does sex and sexuality mean to you; in a society increasingly aware of gender diversity, can you find a place where you belong?

This book isn't just for people with a certain condition: it's for anyone who has felt 'other'; anyone who has felt like they're being left behind; anyone who has questioned their role in society (and what it means if you don't hit universally agreed-upon milestones).

I'll take you through my journey, from carrying tampons, to sitting in an IVF clinic with my bestie, and my ongoing quest to 'fit in', before I realised one thing: it's overrated, my friend!

In fact, I think I was always meant to be born this way.

Sure, I pictured children, picket fences and happily-ever-afters, but I think the 'universe' had bigger plans for me.

A friend once said, 'Ally, the world needs all sorts of mothers. The world needs healers, teachers, educators, storytellers and nurturers.'

I get that now.

Eleven years ago, I decided through a handful of turnaround moments to restart my life. Up until that point, I was a passenger in life, waiting for a well-overdue debt to be paid to me that I was entitled to receive.

In fact, I was owed nothing.

I hadn't been wronged. I wasn't being punished.

But I was going to be challenged. I was going to have to earn my happiness. Becoming a voice for the voiceless was the leap I needed to take. It was my invitation to get off the victim conveyor belt and rejoin life once and for all.

So that is what I did.

By the end of this book, I hope that you are not sitting in an unhappy relationship, that you trust that happiness is waiting for you. If you are living in a body that is disconnected from your heart, that you can learn to embrace it. If you are bursting at the seams to speak your truth, that you find the courage to let some secrets free. And most importantly, if you are trying to fit into a definition of womanhood that feels a little different right now, that you learn to love the perfectly put-together human you are. Because you are damn incredible!

I have become a relentless advocate, who is determined to reduce stigma, challenge taboo, normalise differences (as I'm not a fan of the word 'normal') and flip perspectives on what it means to be a woman in the twenty-first century.

But will I, through writing this book, answer the question that has haunted me for years: 'When will I feel like a woman?'

Thank you for being here.

Ally xo

PART ONE
Unlearning it all

CHAPTER 1

Did you *really* just say the word VAGINA?

After launching my new podcast, *Stigma Shakers*, only a few short months ago, there was one episode when I was smug enough to think, 'This is the one that will skyrocket my followers. This is the episode that will thrust me into the "social media activist" limelight. This is the episode that is going to see my inbox flooded with DMs applauding me for how daring, bold and inspirationally vulnerable I was for pressing "share".'

'OK, Instagram, let's do this!'

Slowly, I saw the odd notification pop up on my iPhone home screen. With my puffed-out boobs, I thought, 'Yeah, Ally, this is catching on like dildos in the Eighties!' So of course, naturally, it was only a matter of time before my Instagram views were going to double, triple, and eventually break the entire internet. OK, that's a *little* extreme, but I did know that I was onto something big, by outing the lingo behind 'solo-pleasure-for-one'.

This episode I was so proud to title, 'Don't Mind If I Do: The Stigma of Masturbation', or should I say, 'M*STURBAT!ON'?

But, let's face it – masturbation and pleasure together remain one of the most radical and taboo topics out there.

Sure, bedroom antics and sexual pleasure are a personal choice – however, are we missing out on a world of exploration when it comes to understanding what makes our bodies feel good?

In this candid podcast episode, we chatted about vagina symbolism, how to welcome lube with open arms, the benefits of self-pleasure, and why our sexual freedom rests in the hands of artificial intelligence.

Immediately, I was shadow-banned, which sounds weirdly sexy and cool and dangerous; how rebellious, but it absolutely isn't. What was my humble crime? I dared to say the word 'vagina', gasp!

Instagram references this 'virtual power' in their Community Guidelines: 'Overstepping these boundaries may result in deleted content, disabled accounts, or other restrictions.'

Woah, what did I do wrong?

Only after removing any associated hashtags and misspelling certain 'risqué' words of a 'restricted nature in accordance with Instagram's Community Guidelines' did I see my engagement increase.

Just when I thought it was safe to talk about vaginas, metadata and the 'algorithm gods' found me. It's really no wonder why punctuation replacements, AKA '#VAG!NA', are one of the few ways to inspire the masses (without being cancelled!).

For now, anyway.

Gosh, even when I've misspelled 'vagina' by accident in this book (#typos), no spelling correction alternative was offered!

Oh, how tragically ironic.

But it wasn't the shadow-ban that left me appealing to my followers (and Instagram) later that night for support.

It was because for most of my life, I have had a shadow-ban of my very own: I have spent a lifetime hiding from the word 'vagina' for reasons that you will understand as you read this book.

And the scary part is, just as I've become ready to lead a life of unapologetic and shame-free living, not only am I late to the party, but perhaps there isn't even a party to go to? Not one that I would be allowed into, anyway.

IS IT SAFE TO COME OUT NOW?

This book, my memoir of missing parts, is a deeply personal (and public) story about living with a rare and hugely taboo medical condition. On each page you turn, you'll learn a bit more about me and my scrappy relationship with relationships, the masterpiece that is my custom-made vagina, and how this body part has influenced how I exist in the world.

You will read my funny anecdotes of how I've announced to first dates, 'Gee, you like my vagina? I made it myself,' and why I am a movement maker and fierce advocate in the world of women's health. You will hear a lot about my womb-less life, and how crippling infertility grief can be.

You hopefully will understand my two different voices: the one that was a fearful and ashamed, broken young woman; and the other, the 'now Ally', who is on a campaign to announce that the only thing normal in this world is difference.

And I am not alone in this, far from it.

Meta has silenced thousands of sex-positive accounts in recent years. Sexual wellness brands, sex educators, activists and sex workers have fallen foul of censorship. Instagram continues to suspend hundreds of high-profile accounts, cutting people off from the communities that keep them safe.

Not only is social media their main source of ethical income, but this social media 'cancel culture' is sending one terrifying message to the world: 'Girls and women, your body is wrong. Don't talk about it. Don't advocate for it. Don't protect it. Don't celebrate it. Don't rally for it.

Don't be proud of it. Don't own it. Don't touch it. Don't learn about it. Don't understand it. Don't feel pain in it. Don't explore it. Don't be honest about it. Don't respect it. Just maybe, don't say anything at all.'

With sexual censorship on the rise, our social media sex educators need a societal shift more than ever! And I consider myself someone who inspires hard conversations when it comes to all things 'below the belt'!

Research commissioned by Bodyform UK, one of the UK's leading menstrual product brands, found that 71 per cent of women don't feel comfortable having open conversations about their bodies, 46 per cent feel there's a stigma around using medical terminology to describe women's anatomy, and only 20 per cent feel comfortable speaking about women's anatomy and bodies with their children.[1]

Further to this, the research study revealed that social media users aren't aware of the censorship, with 85 per cent of Brits not knowing vagina is the most flagged word on Facebook. A further two-thirds (68 per cent) didn't know sharing an educational image of a vulva could get you banned on social media, and 7 in 10 didn't know what shadow-banning was or that it regularly happens.

These stats are alarming, but they aren't the scariest of them all.

Wait for it – this study revealed the top 40 words relating to women's health that are being censored on social media. Please allow me to share: vagina, miscarriage, fibroids, lactation, endometriosis, PMS, sex, infertility, PCOS, orgasm, clitoris, tampon, discharge, boobs, labia, minora, labia majora, vulva, period, period products, dysmenorrhoea, amenorrhoea, puberty, breastfeeding, cervix, bacterial vaginosis, HPV, adenomyosis, colposcopy, panty, undies, vaginal atrophy, menstrual cycle, nipples, UTI, uterus and ... menopause.

---

1 'Vaginas Uncensored: 40 words you can't use', Bodyform: www.bodyform.co.uk/break-taboos/our-campaigns/vagina-uncensored/

As Kristina Cahojova, founder and CEO at Kegg, a US-based technology company that assists with infertility tracking, so perfectly says, 'Women's health is suppressed on social media. It's not because we are violating terms and conditions, it's because of sloppy AI that is flagging us as sex or porn.'

Instagram, what she said.

IT'S A MOVEMENT-Y KIND OF A DECADE

Despite my podcast not breaking the entire internet, I've spent the last 13 years talking about my vagina because, as you'll read, I was born without one. But a little more on that later. As I don't want to be a one-trick vagina pony, I have become an activist, campaigner and 'good vagina sport'. I know what it's like to sit with shame on a daily, if not hourly, basis. And let's be honest – how many stigmas continue to silence the world?

During my research for the *Stigma Shakers* podcast, I wanted to expose the top stigmas we face as a society. Over a cuppa one day with my TV-producer friend Maddie, we teased out our top-10 taboos that cripple so many, including: masturbation, sex work, intersex, grief, gendered health, loneliness, people-pleasing and divorce. Talking about these subjects takes quite the bundle of bravery, I know. I can speak publicly, but this was a first – even for me.

Listening back to certain episodes, it dawned on me how silent we all are.

Sure, we have read bumper-sticker quotes posted from platform to platform, but I am not entirely convinced if this is enough to tackle taboos head-on in the way that we truly need. As a self-confessed stigma shaker and #vag!nawriter, I feel a familiar wave of blame and shame, as I question, 'Has the world really accepted difference?'

Will the world *really* ever see me as a woman, despite not growing a bump for nine months? Will I ever make a name for myself if all I talk about is vaginas? Will I ever feel completely comfortable in my womanly curves if I've never felt like a complete one? Even though I know that having a vagina doesn't make you a woman, even though I know that curves don't make you a woman, at times, I still judge myself by that criteria: it's bullshit. So, I need to call out the bullshit!

I get it.

'Vagina' can be a confronting word.

But isn't my vagina as valid as my eyeball? Or isn't my vagina as valid as my mental health? Or isn't my vagina as important as a working spleen? In saying that, you can live without a spleen – or can you? Anyway, you get what I mean. Because technically, you can live without a vagina. But that's *not* the point.

The point is, our future generations are learning that their body is shameful.

Come on world, we can do better!

Because let's face it, VAGINA is not a dirty word, VAGINA is not shameful, VAGINA should not be taboo, and now's the time to stamp out stigma once and for all.

MY HOLE STORY ISN'T MY (W)HOLE STORY

Then there's the love story between me and myself, and my forever search to find my person who could simply accept 'me'. Not the bad, toxic type of love I experienced in my twenties and thirties, but the type of love that makes you feel like you're 'home'.

Externally, you'd never know that I was born without a womb and a vagina (because the vulva and vagina are two separate parts). And you could say the same about my self-esteem. As a former theatre arts student, I was good at playing the part of 'strong and sexy', but inside, I've always questioned how believable my Oscar-worthy performance in the role of 'woman' came across to others.

I often joke about how my vagina became my biggest career break, and in so many ways, it has been. I've travelled the world as a keynote speaker, stood in front of the camera bearing it all, and even now, this book exists because once my vagina did not.

But sometimes, you've got to put the one-liners aside, because we all know how it feels to be lonely, wondering if a microwave meal-for-one is our ultimate destiny. This memoir is not your average 'Bridget Jones' tell-all exposé, but a really relatable story of how exhausting love can be. But, most importantly, how magical it can feel when you find yourself saying, 'Today, I am really happy,' and totally mean it. It's a rare type of day for so many people, but so is any original love story.

So, now in my early forties, I am finally ready to tell the full and frank story behind the clickbait headlines, 'The Girl Born Without a Vagina', and the struggles we all feel when it comes to loving the skin we are in.

CHAPTER 2

The other sex talk

I was never a happy teenager. I was a dark and moody one, beyond the usual hormonal, spotty prerequisites that come with growth spurts. I was a deep thinker, a deep feeler, and for the most part, I still am. But back then I didn't know it had a name; I didn't know it was depression.

I didn't have the toolkits or strategies to strive for a better day. Being a teenager is hard work. We are trying to answer all the big life questions in one sitting: what career will I take? Who will I marry? How many children will I have? What will love feel like? What will success look like?

What I didn't expect to ask myself was, 'Why haven't I got my first period yet?'

My mum and I have an incredible relationship. You will hear me talk about her a lot. She is so much more than a mother; she is my soulmate. We were designed for each other. I am almost certain that if there is something greater out there, greater than me, they paired us perfectly.

But, despite an unbreakable mother-and-daughter bond, when my mum was prepped for the period conversation, I was awkward, embarrassed and NOT relishing the moment.

As I was approaching my GCSEs, it was about to get really 'real'. From the back of a wardrobe, my mum pulled out a nappy-like, heavy-duty, sling sanitary towel. Nothing could have prepared me for my introduction to womanhood like that did.

Sure, I wasn't 'au fait' with every female product out there, but I figured that a tampon or something just a little smaller would suit my needs.

Nup. Not this time.

I was terrified that after I finished an exam, I would be the girl who stood up to expose a big red bloody stain on my school uniform. So, for 21 days, in every exam, I would sit in what felt like a vintage nappy, courtesy of my mum.

I didn't do too well in my exams, and I never did get a period.

But there was something else that I knew wasn't right.

Something I have never shared with anyone, just you.

The lack of a menstrual cycle was not the reason I had a quiet cause for concern. I learnt a little about vaginas in science class, but a lot from porn. You learn bits here and there, and teenage girls talk a lot about 'things down there', more than our parents would like to know. And in many ways, teens are way better at talking about bits and bobs than adults.

So, I gave it a go.

I tried to masturbate.

I knew where my fingers were *supposed* to go, how to move them and the rhythm they were meant to make.

It was then I knew there was a real problem.

WAS MY WOMANHOOD OVER BEFORE IT EVEN BEGAN?

As teenagers, we read books and magazines that explain how our bodies will change and develop. We learn about sex education and reproduction, awkwardly, in science classes. We wait patiently and eagerly for our first period to arrive. We imagine how we might lose our virginity and the mothers we will become. Being a teenager can be brutal, yet so hopeful and so innocent.

For me, that innocence was soon to be replaced by a discovery that would trigger a life of near misses, self-disgust, bedroom berating and complete sadness.

I will never forget the day the doctor stood by my hospital bed and drew an olive-green curtain around me. My mum sat to my left, holding my hand. There was a nurse to my right, standing just slightly behind my consultant. In one sentence, this doctor, this stranger, changed my life forever.

Using a pencil, he went on to draw a diagram of my reproductive system. I had been admitted for a routine procedure called a laparoscopy, where a small microscope was inserted through my abdomen to investigate what's working, or in my case, not working. Still groggy from the anaesthesia, I was trying to follow the lines of lead, as he outlined a picture of my body.

It wasn't my reaction that hit the silence first, it was my mum's. She clutched her jaw, as though she was trying to control every nerve in her body from exploding. She was crying, but I couldn't understand why.

And then I heard my doctor repeat, 'Alison, we are so sorry to tell you that you have been born without a womb, cervix and vagina.'

No womb.

No cervix.

No vagina.

What the actual fuck?

Decades later, I can talk about this medical jargon on autopilot. I was born with a unique and rare condition called Mayer-Rokitansky-Küster-Hauser syndrome (MRKH).

I am a 1 in 5,000 statistic.

There are two types of MRKH: Type 1, characterised by the absence or underdevelopment of the uterus, cervix and vaginal canal; and Type 2, which includes the key characteristics of Type 1, which in addition, can affect kidney development, skeletal changes, hearing difficulties and even heart abnormalities. According to Imperial College Healthcare NHS Trust,[2] it is estimated that approximately 40 per cent of women with MRKH will have Type 2.

During one of my first medical appointments, it was explained to me that my vagina was roughly the length of a fingernail. My 'dimple', as they commonly call it, was extremely underdeveloped.

It was explained to me that if I wanted to have a penetrative sex life, I would have to 'create' my own vagina.

If I wanted to have a 'normal' sex life and reclaim my female body, I would have to create my very own, custom-made vagina. At the time there were two options: surgery or dilation – and I chose the latter as the less invasive treatment.

Remember, I was 16 years old.

For a long and traumatic nine months, both morning and night, I would insert pink, hard tubes into this fingernail-sized dimple and push hard. Eventually, this routine, which required a white-knuckled grip, would create a vagina.

It physically worked. By the end of nine months – ironically, the time it takes to grow a baby – I had a fully working vagina. Well, kind of. I could have physical sex. I could be penetrated. I could feel pleasure. My vagina, however, was a 'dead-end', so I would never have a period or be able to conceive naturally.

---

2   'Mayer Rokitansky Küster Hauser syndrome (MRKH): Information for patients, relatives and carers', Imperial College Healthcare NHS Trust, February 2019: https://www.imperial.nhs.uk/-/media/website/patient-information-leaflets/childrens-services/disorders-of-sexual-development-and-adolescent-gynaecology/mrkh.pdf

And then there were the emotional repercussions.

Me and my vagina were set never to respect one another or connect for the next 23 years. I had to completely perfect the art of disconnection if I was to survive this trauma.

There is a part of my pre-diagnosis story I never share.

There was a moment – a crucial coming-of-age moment – before my sixteenth birthday, when I knew I was different.

On a family holiday to Greece, with my best friend at the time, my mum and her partner, I tried to have sex with a barman. Since all my friends were losing their virginity, it felt like the thing to do.

I met him at a tacky disco-tech in the early hours of the morning and we fell into a holiday romance. He was beautiful. I actually thought I was in love with him at the time. Of course I did. Gosh, I would have moved continents for him back then. In fact, I wrote him a letter professing my plans. I never, ever heard back.

Despite every consensual effort to lose my virginity, his penis was not making any headway with my non-existent vagina.

I felt embarrassed, confused and yuck.

Not because I tried to have sex, but because I couldn't.

In popular culture, so much emphasis is placed on the day you lose your virginity. This is, however, another side of the story. The unsexy truth is that not everyone can, not everyone will.

This isn't something that any version of 'the talk' will tell us.

I WILL NEVER FORGET THE DAY

After my diagnosis, my dad was the first person that Mum and I phoned. I could see her lean like a deadweight onto the phone box in the corridor, just steps from my head. Her expression was like she was telling someone close to her that someone had died. Her face revealed a grief that I hadn't seen before.

Her lips barely moved, and her breathing was slow. Her eyes were closed, she slowly rolled her head from side to side. In some ways, something had died. Perhaps she was grieving, even then.

Grieving the grandchildren she assumed I would give her, grieving my future as a woman, my happiness. We can so easily assume that everything in life turns out one way. We assume that girls have periods, girls will have babies, girls will be 'normal'.

Rarely do we prepare ourselves for the unimaginable.

Gosh, my dad was, and is, a brave man. We so often recall the moments of our past as daughters, where our mum is at the rescue. But dads do it hard too. They absorb the same hard-hitting news, yet somehow, they are expected to cope differently. And in many ways, they do.

I will always remember his stoicism and strength, so that I would feel those things too.

So that I would feel hopeful, capable and supported.

There was, however, only so far he could go. The next part, I would have to do alone.

I remember, the hospital ward felt so cold. The walls were a greyish green, and there was a tiny, locked balcony in the corner of my room. I am pretty sure I saw the odd cigarette butt on the ledge, probably from the anxious girl before me who may also have had to make a vagina.

As I settled into my three-day stay at the London hospital, I unpacked two tubes of Pringles, a heap of celebrity magazines, my CD player and a few clothes.

After all, I was there to create my vagina. How could I know what to pack for that?

WAS I LOSING MY VIRGINITY ... WITH MYSELF?

I will never forget the position I had to get into to force a dilator into my body – flat on my back with my feet on the floor and my knees apart. This position still haunts me. Whenever I get into that position in yoga or even lie on my back, that time resurfaces – an incredibly vulnerable part of my journey.

A nurse sat on the end of the bed, directing me on how to hold and insert the dilator. She would explain how much pressure to apply, the tilt that would be most effective – and if 'my knuckles turned white', I was doing it correctly.

We started on the smallest dilator first. Over time, you 'graduate' to larger dilators, which were made out of Pyrex. I was so cared for, but no amount of smiling was going to penetrate (excuse the pun) this horrific situation that I was experiencing as a child.

My memories of the staff didn't make me sick.

It was the fact that I was losing what felt like my virginity ... with an object, alone and in tears.

Quiet, palpable, sobbing salty tears were all I could muster.

Making a vagina is a little like losing weight; the first few days, or weeks, you will see big results, fast. After that, the progress feels sluggish.

Crafting my own vagina was far from glamorous. Unlike the fancy ones with jewels and diamonds, mine was more akin to a basic flat-packed, pre-ordered-looking thing. There was no colour chart, assembly guide or how-to diagram – just me and a bag of tubes. I held onto dilators just as firmly as I held onto my hopes for a 'normal' sex life, normality and womanhood.

I don't remember much more, other than one moment that explained the gravity of what I had just done to my body.

Walking through London Paddington station, on my way home, I was struggling to keep up with my mum, who was sprinting to the train.

I couldn't sprint. I couldn't even walk.

And just like that, I was on my knees.

Bereft.

Crying.

Gasping for breath.

The pain I had experienced, the exposure of my body, the disgust I felt as I recalled inserting objects into my body, was simply too much. Now I can put it into words – it all felt like an act of self-abuse.

With hundreds of commuter onlookers, I was crying in the centre of London.

Weekly, I would go to the village chemist to buy KY Jelly (lube!), and I would be upstairs in the family home making my vagina, while my family pretended that I wasn't.

Those three, solitary days in hospital were like a dynamite bomb. The impact, the devastation and emotional casualties were mine to treat for the next 20 years of living.

Recently, at an upmarket café in London, sipping fancy coffee and picking away at cheesecake (because, eating disorder 'recoveree'), I explained to a new friend my old 'vaginal dilation wins'.

It was through this candid chat that I gave her a free pass to ask me any questions she had, which perhaps before, she felt too weirded out by. So she did.

'Ally, can you pee?'

'Ally, do you look like a Barbie doll down there?' (Trust me, she is not alone in this query!)

'Ally, have you experienced orgasms?'

I took a breath, smiled at her honesty, and replied:

'Yes, I can pee, out of my urethra, which I was born with. I have the complete vulva package.'

'I do not look like a Barbie doll down there. Externally, you'd never know.'

'I love orgasms. I mean, who doesn't? Sometimes it happens, sometimes it doesn't. Like for so many, orgasms are never a given!'

I am not the first person to take a stab at dismantling a version of 'womanhood'.

Some might say that we're living in a 'progressive' world, while others may symbolise womanhood against the fake and flatness of a Barbie doll (or a similar branded item).

Does Barbie have a typical-looking vulva?

Where are her stretch marks and dangly boobs?

We see she has no vagina, so is this on purpose too?

Are we meant to be benchmarking our 'womanhood Richter scale' against a hole, or is it safer to show no difference?

Is the iconic Barbie doll an outdated symbol of womanhood, or is she perfectly spot on?

Is Barbie a 'child-free' icon?

The thing is, Barbie, in fact, never married or had babies.

That's because Ruth Handler, the creator of Barbie, did not want to reinforce the idea that young girls should aspire only to marriage and motherhood.

So, while I do not look like Barbie 'down there', perhaps we are a little alike after all.

Still, back in the late 1990s, I was nowhere near discovering my own definition of womanhood.

I am mortified (and profoundly apologetic) that I explained to my family how far I pushed the dilator into my body. I could tell, because my KY Jelly lubricant acted as my vaginal 'spirit level'. It was the only way I could physically track progress. But I wasn't sharing this news because I was proud, it was because I was drunk and in shock. After all, if I was tipsy I couldn't feel, which was the last thing I wanted to do.

My family was not overlooking my drinking habits, but nor could they tame the unthinkable. It's hard to know how to prepare for trauma when we haven't been to that place before. So, my family, while perturbed at my brazen ability to humour the unimaginable, were simply following my lead.

Could she be OK with all of this?

Maybe it's not so devastating after all?

Perhaps happiness is measured differently with a daughter navigating MRKH?

Geez, they did their absolute best.

But to be honest, they didn't stand a chance.

Because I was determined to self-destruct. I was determined to undo, unravel, dismantle and destroy any chance at being a happy, healthy and hopeful teen. I was a tornado that was going to demolish everything in my path. And what makes it worse is that I was good at it.

And what really made it worse ... is that I enjoyed it.

CHAPTER 3

Grieving womanhood as a child

I was never a popular student at school, but I was never lingering on my own.

I was a 'groupie-grazer'; friends with everyone but I never wanted to stand out. Which is quite ironic, given that I wanted to become a famous Hollywood actress.

I am still proudly sharing how I was Sandy in a production of *Grease* at school, an accolade that I am unlikely ever to drop, despite it being incredibly uncool of me to keep sharing it.

I loved to perform and write. I loved using my imagination and creating intelligent work. I loved the idea of magic and fantasy. Once, I tried to be a goth, despite me failing at black lipstick. After that, I was a hippy. I tried anything and everything to find my spot.

But sometimes, individuality *is* our spot.

Being a deep thinker back then, however, was like fire and gasoline after my MRKH diagnosis. Previously, I had dabbled in self-harm. Well, quite a bit. But this earth-shattering diagnosis gave me the ultimate permission to fuck up.

The scars on my arms and boobs tell *that* story.

I would self-harm, not for attention (though that's an absolutely valid cry for help) – I was harming myself because I couldn't find the valve to let out the red mist that was suffocating me.

I was angry yet silent. I was desperate and defeated. I wanted to belong, but I was so lonely. I wanted to reverse everything that had happened to me, while praying for a quick exit from this reality that I was trying to accept.

I would cut myself in the bath, in school toilets and even before occasions I was looking forward to. On the second night of my Sandy school performance, my mum wanted to pass me a top through my bedroom door.

It was then she clocked my unhealed and scabby cuts.

She was devastated. I was mortified and guilty that I had let her down.

We didn't talk about it that night. Instead, I heard her cry proudly in the audience as they applauded. But she was applauding differently. She was applauding my bravery.

She was so proud of my strength, and yet so grief-stricken that a girl who did so well was so brokenly brave. She tried to help but I wasn't ready because I needed to break.

And if there was a way to break, I found it.

It's not uncommon for acts of self-harm to be coupled with eating disorders. Only months before my MRKH diagnosis, I was starting to count calories obsessively. I was starting to create eating rituals that, in ways, still exist today. Something in me just knew something wasn't right, but I had no idea what it was; a sadness that I couldn't explain.

I can't eat carbs before sugary treats, and remain alert to old habits slipping back in. I am pleased to say, while a negative relationship with food never completely leaves us, I am not governed, obsessed or consumed with not being 'thin' enough.

Back then, I would only allow myself 400 calories a day.

I did try bulimia, but honestly, I did half the job: I could binge but not purge. I was a 'lazy bulimic' who couldn't 'guarantee' removal of the consumed count.

So, starvation was my go-to and proven method of rapid weight loss. I would be so tired, and cold, yet energised by hunger. I was winning at life because I was failing at womanhood. Unlike self-harming, I had no problem with demonstrating how successful I was at abstaining from food.

It was a weird, and self-confessed, celebration of control.

As a former anorexic, my mum saw the signs. And she said all the right things. But nothing was going to dent the sides of how fixated I was on destroying myself. How determined I was to validate why I was dirty, incomplete, and why I was never going to be enough.

I felt like a defective freakshow.

I have come to realise that, throughout my teens, twenties and early thirties, I liked to feel instant relief. Sitting in pain was my 'stuck at sea' moment of desperation, so avoidance was key.

I have now learnt that there is no shortcut to acceptance; no B-road or hard shoulder to park on. To avoid the bright lights of an emotional pile-up, we must drive through tough things slowly.

But what happens when you feel like your life is over before it has even had a chance to begin?

It was going to get a whole lot worse before it got better.

IT'S A FAMILY THING

When something happens to one family member, it typically happens to them all. That's the magic of a close family. While my family couldn't understand every thought I was thinking, they offered me limitless love. I have always been so close with both of my parents, and while some conversations go unspoken about the 'birds and the bees', it was a tricky time for any of us to hide from.

It's not uncommon for children and their parents to have two-way awkwardness around sex talk. For them, sitting in the doctor's office, listening to my 'vagina-making' options, was hard. Not because they were prudish, but because they were in shock. However, never once was I silenced. Never once was I made to feel ashamed or embarrassed; I was doing a pretty good job at that on my own.

They would often ask me how I was, and how my treatment was going. They were following my lead. They would comfort me by showering me with compassion, patience and leniency. I got away with more. Just months before my diagnosis, I got a tattoo on my hip (a baby cherub of all things). Neither of them knew about this random ink stain on my skin, but once it was revealed post-diagnosis, their annoyance was heavily downplayed.

My mum had talked to me about sex once, and the difference between sex and intimacy. I remember it vividly, and how she wanted me to know that sex is sacred and protection is a must! She wanted me, and my brother, to understand that sex is healthy and can be the perfect act between two people who love one another. If only I believed her at the time.

Because sex, for me, started with plastic tubes.

Not sacred, not love, not 'normal'.

I often wonder, if I had a daughter and she was diagnosed with MRKH, what would I say?

First, I would want her to know that she is loved.

That her body is not incomplete, defective or freakish. I would walk with her through each scary step and trauma cry, with compassion and freedom to feel. I would want her to know that while her future may look different, it can still be full. That her body is perfect. That she can choose to create a vagina, or she can choose to wait. That her worth is not measured by her anatomy. That she must accept love, and nothing less, in a partner.

That her courage is her greatest asset.

And again, that she is loved.

THE ART OF DISCONNECTION

As children, we are taught at school, through pop culture, family soap operas and general chit-chat, that biology works. We, as teenagers, are sat down in a science class and given a sexual reproduction tutorial. We are offered diagrams and low-budget explanatory videos of what anatomy we have, how contraception works (usually with the aid of a banana or some phallic-shaped vegetable), and what happens when a boy and girl have sex with each other.

I didn't tune out, but I don't remember all that much to tune in to. We are often taught that the typical road to womanhood is through a rite of passage to parenthood and partnership. We are taught that a penis goes in a vagina. Sometimes these vaginas bleed, and if they don't, a baby is on the way.

This insane simplification is all we had to model our futures on. So, when all these things don't take place, then what?

It's hard to imagine how three days in a hospital ward 'making' my vagina can do so much damage. After all, what is 72 measly hours? It's not like I hadn't been exposed to difficulty before. I had witnessed my parents survive their divorce, my mum had discovered sobriety and I was a practising self-harmer and eating disorder devotee.

Although I had only self-harmed once prior to my diagnosis, I knew it came with instant relief. As warped as that sounds, self-harm felt like letting a little steam out of the pressure cooker; the steam being a messy mind.

When I was admitted to the London hospital for my three-day inpatient vaginal dilation treatment, something happened to me.

Something devastating, and so incredibly sad, took place in those brief but life-altering moments. In fact, just writing these words makes my arms feel heavier. Like the memory of what I had to do back then is quicksand for the soul. It's a drowning feeling. It's grief.

The teenage years are already fraught with confusion: who am I? What sexuality am I? Who will I become? Where will I live? What type of mother will I be? Our curiosity to predict our future turns into the centre of our friendship conversations. I had no reason to believe that I wouldn't be able to have sex or become a parent.

It's a given, isn't it?

As young adults, our formative years are partly responsible for learning our worth. We are untangling our ideals, values and morals. We are rebellious enough to discover our boundaries, and remorseful enough to right our wrongs. Our dreams don't feel like dreams back then, they feel like possibilities on the other side of 'growing up'. In fact, I don't think we ever doubt our future as teens; it's not a case of if but when, at that age.

So, when a truck slams into your emotional pathways, and destroys everything you thought you knew or could become, it's impossible to know how to recover from that. I didn't have yoga back then, or a handful of wise and insightful friends. I had caring and loving parents, but they followed my lead. I gave them reason to believe it was all going to be fine.

I was a wannabe actress, after all.

A CRASH COURSE IN SHAME

When you lie on your back, eyes wide open, knees apart, and force an object into your body, you are learning what shame feels like. You are learning to couple pain with progress, sadness with success, and intimacy with inanimate objects. It is no wonder why, for much of my life, I equated sex with disgust. I didn't have shame for my sexual partners, but I did for myself.

When I lost my virginity at the age of 17, it felt fiddly, but good. I was quietly happy that my vagina was 'in good working order', and hopefully, the man I had chosen was none the wiser. Because it did feel like a job. It felt like part of the treatment plan, or process, to this place called womanhood. The next day I looked into the mirror, hoping to see a different person staring back at me; confident and initiated into the world of sex.

I am not naive. I know that 'first-time' encounters are nothing like the movies. These encounters are often clumsy, slippery, haphazard and giggly. While I had experienced sexual activity with real humans, I had already made up my mind about sex.

For me, sex was nothing more than a jigsaw puzzle. If that bit fits that bit, and that bit goes in that bit, and if you move your body that way, and make the sounds this way, it's sex. But it certainly wasn't sacred.

To dilate, you need to have the ability to zone out. If you are going to master pain and shame, you need to disconnect your body from your mind, your worth. There was no other way for me. The only problem was, I never reconnected ... until one night, in the distant future, I did.

MY SECRET WASN'T MINE

I was only months away from starting to study for A-levels when I left the hospital. Some knew about it, and some didn't, including teachers and students. I had to take a week off school for the laparoscopic surgery, which first uncovered MRKH. At first, returning to school felt effortless ... until it wasn't.

As sixth-formers, we were asked to dress in formal clothes: trousers, shirt, blazer or something remotely presentable. I think they were trying to prepare us for the grown-up world, and in many ways, I thought I was quite mature.

Perhaps it was my arty, deep side that gave me a sense of profound thinking. As someone hovering around anorexia, my trousers – wonderfully baggy – made me look tall and svelte. The problem was, hunger generally catches up. After months of living off 400 calories a day, I was cold and tired. Despite starvation boosting my adrenaline, I was consumed with food patterns: mealtimes on the dot, calories counted, concave stomach check, and wondering if I'd ever eat a chip again.

It's not uncommon for anorexics to swing the other way: to binge. As you know, I tried the bulimic thing, but it wasn't the right disorder for me. Not only did I hate being sick, I thought the process lacked guarantee. How can you truly determine that it would all come up? Wouldn't the calories cling to your inner muscles and fatty deposits? Tragic thought processing.

Instead, I began bingeing without the release – overeating and overeating until I wanted to be sick but couldn't.

My mum knew what I was doing as someone who has experienced eating disorders herself. It's not hard to spot when you've walked in those dark shoes. My sudden weight gain was also evident. I went from wearing fitted blazers at school to baggy jumpers because I was self-conscious of my changing body.

After drama class, my teacher pulled me aside. She wanted to know why I was not conforming to the dress code. All I could say was, 'I hate the body that I am being forced to live within.' I can't even remember how she responded.

Not long after, I dropped out of school at the age of 17. At the time, I was studying drama and English literature. I wanted to become a writer. I wanted to work in the arts and media industry and be surrounded by people like me, who love to think and feel deeply.

I knew I had the ability to be successful, but so often, I would find myself sitting alone. I felt like I was segregated from my friends, who were talking about period pains and first-time sexual encounters. I no longer belonged there. In fact, I didn't belong anywhere. Only in the darkness that became my greatest familiarity and comfort.

My secret was not so secret anymore.

Like my art of physical detachment, I had also learnt how to detach myself from my reality. Here's the funny thing: if we don't understand the magnitude of a situation, if we can't comprehend it, we cannot treat it any differently to a tooth filling. Or I didn't.

I had no idea what was happening to me, so, in some ways, I didn't try to avoid sharing it (which, I know, is incredibly conflicting). How can someone know sadness, but not know its cause? Our identity, as humans, is very bloody complex, especially after trauma.

My mental health was in rapid decline and my sense of self-hatred was all I could think about. No one blamed me for my behaviour. I was breaking and no one seemed able to help me. No one knew how to counsel the teenager who had no vagina.

I WAS A PRO AT DESTRUCTION

I believe we are all born with a psyche blueprint. I believe that, like architectural drawings, we have a rough layout of the person we are. Some people have the foundations of depression, anxiety and low self-esteem. Some people have optimism, positivity, confidence and limitless self-belief. Some foundations blur, and others are defined by skill sets, abilities and talents. Of course, this is only a draft; a blueprint that can be tweaked with outside influence, therapists, life-changing moments, self-awareness and perception.

But it's there.

As someone who has always been a deep feeler and massive over-analyser, it's easy for me to get intense. And that's not always the perfect formula. I recently asked a friend rhetorically, 'Would you trade your insight if it meant the deep, dark days were not so dark?' Would we trade our favourite quality for a worse one, if it meant the worse one wouldn't hit so hard?

See, it's all based on polarisation.

A bit like eating disorders and self-harm, there are no half-measures to how to experience feeling or, in many cases, stunt it. While I have spent nearly a decade in therapy, embracing spirituality and surrounding myself with 'real' humans, sometimes 'fucking up' seems so much more familiar than 'healing'.

I didn't just dabble in destructive behaviour after my MRKH diagnosis, I perfected it. I felt somehow safe in the predictability of negative feelings. I became trauma's most committed subscriber; give me a razor blade, a sad song, a bad man, and let me work my magic.

Was I trying to feel something?

Was I punishing myself?

Was I confirming what a worthless piece of shit I was?

If I am not a woman, what does it matter how I implode?

I often wonder: was my blueprint to be someone who would always struggle with worth because of my MRKH diagnosis or despite it? Regardless, I made a pact with myself: Ally, you are going to make damn sure that you find the most dangerous situations, experience the pain you deserve and never take up any more room in a person's life than they offer you.

Take what you get, because you don't deserve any more.

I'd love to say I only carried this mindset for a number of months or years, but I carried it for over a decade. I'm just grateful it wasn't forever. Today, thanks to the events you'll read about in the following chapters, I know that I'm here to do more than suffer.

Now, it's impossible to imagine torturing myself as I did, day after day. That's the funny thing about shame – it can warp your perception of every aspect of life.

CHAPTER 4

Playing a part

After I left school, I lost the identity of a schoolgirl and entered an adult world.

The truth is, not only had I perfected the art of disconnection, I had become a really great liar. I would memorise the names of contraceptive pills so that, if any of my sexual partners asked, I could spin off a line that we were protected. If a girlfriend asked for a tampon I'd say, 'Sorry, I'm not on!' (I've never quite understood the slang for menstrual cycles).

With a faint love of acting left in me, my next tactic was to 'play the part' of a happy human. After all, acting is easy, right? If I could play the role of a 'woman', I would step into the shoes of a person I was craving to be. Was it escapism and denial? Massively. But at the time, I was willing to give anything a go!

When I'd go out to pick up guys in bars, I would call myself 'Sarah'. My alias, Sarah, was a successful actress, who was excited to get married and have children. Sarah was vivacious, sexy and confident. Sarah didn't give a shit about life. That was until my step-grandmother found me in bed, on two separate occasions, with men from the apartment block.

I had gone to stay with my step-grandmother in Australia, after I was clearly not coping in England any longer.

I needed an escape plan. I needed to run.

Months before my MRKH diagnosis, my mum and I were due to travel to Australia together, to visit our family. My mum had grown up in Sydney and left in her early twenties because of her own sense of 'unbelonging', trauma and loss.

As soon as our flight tickets were bought, I felt instant relief. I was going to the land down under, where I would continue making my vagina. At this point, I only had one month to go and then I would feel 'normal', or so I thought.

I was looking forward to spending time with my mum – however, she never made it on that trip. Just weeks before we were due to fly, my brother was involved in a severe and life-threatening motorcycle accident. The accident meant that my mum needed to stay in the UK to care for him. Instead, I would stay with my step-grandmother in Sydney – a grandparent I had met once, briefly, in England.

Despite the last-minute plan, I was hopeful.

Perhaps this would be the place that would reset my trauma? The problem was, I wasn't going as myself. I was going to Australia to pretend to be someone else; any version of myself who wasn't broken.

Before we can acknowledge – and begin to heal – our pain, we first become an actress. We learn how to act OK. We practise our lines, rehearse our better days and smile on cue. It's almost a brief interlude before the big shit gets real. So, that's what I did.

The problem is, you soon lose track of where the truth ends and the façade begins. And, sometimes, reality slaps you in the face exactly when you don't want it to.

I COULDN'T SHAKE SELF-HARM

Australia was a tricky place to self-harm because ... sleeves. Australia's climate doesn't bode well for self-harmers because, unless you are planning on overheating daily, your skin is no longer yours to hide.

I was also living in a house that wasn't my own, under the watchful eye of my step-grandmother. That meant I had to modify my behaviour. I didn't have the tools I needed to self-harm, so I chose starvation as my mode of self-destruction. I smoked constantly. I dyed my hair. Occasionally, I changed my name (again!).

It didn't, however, hide everything about me.

After I lost my virginity, I was pretty much 'sex ready', with only two months to go before my official 'vagina graduation' deadline! It's not unusual to hear that people with MRKH go through subsequent promiscuity. In some ways, we are 'testing out' our new-found body part. We are making sure that we are 'desired' as a woman and that we 'can do the sex' like the other girls.

For me, I had an extra goal: to never, ever go back to dilators ever again.

The fact is, advice has varied over the years about scheduling vaginal dilation into a weekly planner. But in sexless spells, upkeep isn't a bad thing to offer some peace of mind. However, having a healthcare professional's expert advice is always the first point of call for anyone in this situation.

For me, dilation was never going to enter my life again. I would make sure that sex was always available if it meant I would never have to do that 'thing' to myself again. And Australia was not going to rock this plan.

One night, I snuck out of the apartment and joined one of these men at a nearby theatre that he was managing. It was insane and exciting. We skulked in with booze and a bad attitude. As we proceeded to have sex on the back row of the empty theatre, I will never, ever forget his words as he tried to enter me: 'I feel like there's a blockage, Ally.'

We can all recall the sentences that stick to and shake us.

He was absolutely right.

There was a blockage. This blockage was an unfinished vagina.

I felt disgusted – and determined.

There was only one thing to do: 'Next time you dilate, Ally, push even harder. Push till your eyes fill with tears, until your hand hurts and you get that damn vagina finished. And self-harm. You need to do that too, otherwise you will go unpunished for your broken, incomplete self.'

LIVERPOOL, THE CITY THAT NEARLY KILLED ME

For the final two weeks of Australia, my mum did fly out – to be with me and take me home. She had promised to walk with me through the streets of Sydney and she lived up to that promise.

It didn't escape either of us how similar our journeys were. My mum had also fled her home country, to leave an identity that didn't feel right.

Like me, she was on her own escape mission to find love, safety and understanding. And here she was, making amends with her own past, to help me with mine. I guess we all believe that changing our geography will help us heal. In many ways it can, but when you are escaping yourself, there is nothing a compass or mileage will do to remedy a broken way of life.

Seeing your daughter destroy her worth couldn't have been easy for either of my parents, but they never abandoned me. Their love was probably what kept me from ever going too far.

Somehow ... somehow, after returning from Australia, I went back to college, where I got an A-level in English literature. I was due to also graduate with an A-level in psychology, but let's just say, I lost my 'homework'.

My mum can tell that story. I was working as a part-time civil servant processing paperwork for the unfolding 'mad cow disease' crisis. Literally, every piece of paper had been splattered with blood, from the slaughterhouses that were responsible for a nationwide cull.

Out of the blue, I got a phone call on my teeny-tiny Nokia mobile phone. My college bestie at the time had applied to study at Liverpool Hope University, so I decided to give it a random shot. I didn't think, with one C grade in the bag, I was ever going to get a place at university, but through the clearing process, I had a place, if I wanted it.

Sure? That's what people do, right? They go to university and make their family proud. Three months later, I was on the motorway to Liverpool, where I secured a spot in a student village. I honestly felt that this was going to be the turnaround moment, where I would get my graduate degree in theatre studies, and become a famous actress, or writer, or, better still, both!

In Liverpool, I raised my stakes and amped up the danger zone.

Here's the thing, university is not the best place for people who are committed to excess. University is not a great place for people who are unaware of their boundaries when it comes to bargain-priced booze.

Every day, I would wake up feeling remorseful, hungover and hating myself. With maybe one proud lecture under my belt, I would celebrate with pints of cider, bags of peanuts, cheesy chips and boxed white wine. I lived off toasties, cigarette smoke and bad-boy crushes. I laughed the loudest, was quoted the funniest, and sometimes, I even managed to look remotely attractive as I stumbled through student unions and the bars of Liverpool.

I was still, however, playing a part.

Was I living my life or destroying it?

It has taken me a long time to truthfully recall this part of my story. Even in writing this book, I've hovered back and forth on how much to share and whether I can face these feelings. This is one of those terrifying moments as a writer, where you know you are crossing out of your comfort zone – in the name of honesty and breaking down stigma.

It's not that I am ashamed of what happened in Liverpool, but I want to protect the pain of others who love me. Whether you know me or not, it's not easy to read, but this is my story and I want to forgive myself.

I know my people will understand that in order to demonstrate our recovery, we must tell the story of that which nearly broke us.

I DIDN'T WANT TO DIE, I JUST DIDN'T KNOW HOW TO LIVE

My lowest moment started with a bad date. Another bad choice. Another morning-after when I hated my own actions. I had been 'saved' from the date by my closest friend at university, Vicky, who had sent a taxi to the guy's house to collect me, after I called her from his bathroom, vomiting and crying.

Vicky was so kind to me. She was compassionate, safe and unwavering in her loyalty. She was the type of person I wanted to be. And she never, ever stopped showing up for me. She was the type of friend I didn't think I deserved.

By this point, she knew a lot about my condition, MRKH, but I hated her seeing more evidence of my failings. Vicky was waiting when the taxi brought me back to the student village, relieved and equally enraged that I put myself in such a dangerous position.

So was I.

How far was I prepared to take my grief?

Why couldn't I shake the memories of me hurting my body with tubes?

Why did my hands have to smell of KY Jelly and me?

Why couldn't I be born a 'proper' woman?

A week later, Vicky and I had gone back to my flat after a night watching *Billy Elliot* at the cinema. I loved that film. I played (and still do) Stephen Gately's title song, 'I Believe', on repeat. As she crashed on my bed, I sat on my en-suite shower floor staring at grooves between the bathroom tiles. I felt calm, even with the music blaring, listening to a song that made me feel so desperate, when in fact it was a song all about hope. Actually, I am listening to it now.

I selected my harm object of choice.

I clasped.

I stood up.

I placed my left wrist on the side of the basin, palm facing up.

I took a deep breath.

With my right hand, I started hurting my left.

At first, I didn't cut deep enough.

So I tried again.

The blood started to pour.

Then Vicky woke up, turned the music off and saved my life.

PART TWO

Boys, booze and bingeing

CHAPTER 5

Self-destruction became my hobby

I didn't want to die that day at university; I just didn't know how to live. For this reason, I went a little softer. A part of me didn't want it to be a 'forever' decision. I didn't go to the hospital, but I bandaged myself up and knew that something had to change. Unlike my previous self-harm episodes, this time I wanted to be 'found'. Then again, perhaps I didn't. Standing over a sink with a bloody wrist, seeing the expression of shock on Vicky's face, I wondered if I had taken this too far.

Some memories you cannot 'unsee' and possibly never truly resolve. I'd never want anyone else to walk in my shoes, but I do believe that night in the bathroom was one of life's little junctions I needed to arrive at.

By this point, I didn't know what I was grieving anymore. I couldn't determine if I was sad or disgusted. I wasn't sure if my behaviour was a product of making my vagina or my disgust at allowing the men I slept with to underappreciate it.

Every night in Liverpool, I was either drunk or hungover. I would stare at the cute boys I didn't feel worthy of being with. My skinny jeans became tighter as the nights of cheesy chips scoffed in backstreet pizza joints caught up with me. I stopped going to lectures and submitting coursework.

It's crazy how a routine of negative behaviour can become a familiar pattern. When I was spiralling, I felt steady. When I was self-sabotaging, I felt soothed. When I was failing my degree or falling down the stairs drunk, I felt lighter. I didn't need to ease any boredom, because I was consumed with confusion. I didn't need to sleep, because I wasn't ever alert enough to care.

I was becoming a pro at pissing my life up the wall. And here I felt safe. This pain I could do. With every regret or screwed-up decision I made, I was remorseful of the one before. So, I gave myself absolute permission to keep forgiving my behaviour as a reward: booze, boys and bingeing. The ultimate cocktail for a person on a mission to find rock bottom.

IT'S NOT LIKE I DIDN'T TRY

Today, I see 'mini meltdowns' as an act of self-care – but it's all about not going too far. A calculated unravelling can be the perfect way for control freaks, like me, to let some air out of the tyres. It happens to me every six months or so, at the end of a stressful period of work when my work–life balance has gone crazy. I'll cry – a lot! I'll feel the urge to drink a little too much. I'll text an ex. I'll start to make some questionable decisions.

The difference is, I don't drop over the edge. I also don't beat myself up because I'm not coping well enough and not being perfect. If there's one thing I've learnt, it's that it's a vicious spiral; you hate yourself for starting to struggle and so you spiral faster. Self-judgement is fuel for self-sabotaging behaviour.

Nowadays, I welcome a crash rather than fear one, because what is the worst that can happen if I admit to a difficult day? Today, I embrace – and have treatment for – the bouts of depression I experience. Because of this, I can welcome a meltdown and soothe it in a healthier way. I watch out for the red flags so I have ample time to prepare: a phone call scheduled with my bestie, a lean work schedule, zero booze and time to be quiet. If these don't work, an SOS to my therapist. It's all about smoothing the spiral sooner.

In my twenties, however, I wasn't as self-aware. This isn't a judgement on myself; I just didn't have the tools I've learnt since then. My fellow university students were young, like me, and busy working through their own angst and turmoil. There was always someone to drink with; to escape with; to sleep with.

Back then, even though every day was unpredictable and desperate, I didn't realise I was in the thick of something. I thought I was outsmarting and outrunning the worst that could possibly happen – people really seeing me! My friend having to rescue me from a strange man's bathroom, apparently, wasn't enough. Dismantling my choice of self-harm apparatus daily wasn't enough. Failing my university degree wasn't enough.

But something did wake me up.

The same friend who found me during my suicide attempt, a regular saviour and fixer-upper, went home for the weekend. It was the first time since I started uni that she had left. Had I really placed so much of my faith on a person that being alone was too unpalatable to bear?

In a momentary fresh-headed perspective, I made an appointment with the university counsellor and explained to her that I was 'struggling' (erm, understatement). I told her that I was feeling down, out of control, and I didn't know how to find my way back.

She prescribed me antidepressants and sent me on my way. Now, I am a HUGE advocate for medication in order to treat depression. If a form of medication eases the burden to allow for clarity to come through, yep, I am all for a prescription. I think healing requires an emotional entourage – a combo of friends, practices, therapists, strategies and resets.

Unfortunately, I only had these pills to help me. I wasn't aware that, for me, a pill would only be a plaster if I didn't make it part of a deeper programme of treatment. Without talk therapy, a healthier lifestyle and a real sense of purpose, a pill wasn't going to remotely touch the sides.

Looking back, I can see that my truth was really starting to hit home – the truth of how I 'made' myself a woman. Symptoms of post-traumatic stress disorder (PTSD) were starting to appear – vivid dreams, flashbacks and an overactive nervous system, which caused me to flare up with anger, sadness and despair.

Not only was I coming to terms with my diagnosis, but I was coming to terms with how I was 'coming to terms with it'. At that point, I didn't know anyone else with MRKH (which is why, years later, I started a support group for other women). I had no guidebook for how to react or behave at this rare, but not so rare, diagnosis.

Some say an MRKH diagnosis isn't related to PTSD. Some would say that it's a difficult reality, but not everyone arrives at the place I did. There is actually no right, or dare I say wrong, way to cope, because we are all messy and complex humans in search of answers. I can say, from experience, few women emerge emotionally unscathed from this diagnosis or the treatment.

At the time of my diagnosis, I hadn't even taken out a phone contract, but I had made my own vagina. The extremity of this statement is as warped as it is literal.

After collecting my antidepressants from the pharmacy, I went back to the student village and called my dad. I'd usually phone both my parents when I had a bad day, typically my mum first. This time, I happened to call my dad – a loving and practical man, who would do anything to protect, love and shield me. For him, the fact that I was now on medication was rock bottom. How contrasting our versions of rock bottom can be!

Days later, I was passing my clothes and bedding through my dorm window as we loaded up the car. I was leaving Liverpool and returning to our home town, no longer a university student, but a university dropout.

I don't remember trying to fight my dad's suggestion that it was time to go home, but I did have regrets. The saddest part of my Liverpool unravelling wasn't the disgusting man feeding me gin for breakfast, or the harm I inflicted upon myself. It was never saying goodbye to Vicky.

It took me another 25 years to find her. Eventually I gave her the apology she deserved, and the thank-you that I forgot to give her for saving me.

FALLING OFF A BAR STOOL GOT ME THE JOB

If you turn a bar stool upside down, it will fit perfectly on the base of another – this is what I learnt over the next few months. It wasn't a lot, but it was something – life's discoveries that make you feel like you're winning, after one big failure at higher education.

I discovered the trick while propping up the bar at the Anchor, a student bar in the centre of Reading. This pub would become my regular and eventually my employer. I became friends with the locals and drank cider 'with a dash of black' on the daily.

I had come back to Reading, my hometown in Berkshire, but I had no intention of coming back to heal. My parents were possibly hoping for a different outcome, but a change of location wasn't going to cure this. As I've previously alluded to, geography cures little when we don't do the work. Our emotions don't have an inbuilt GPS. Our stories, traumas, bad days and wounds are blind to where we are – they just travel within us until we are ready for the perfect view.

With my savings dwindling and my career as a lawyer, writer or actress firmly parked, I needed to get work, fast. One thing I have always been, even when I had no desire to be a university graduate, is a worker.

My unwavering work ethic is a credit to my parents, who taught my brother and me that nothing comes for free and being a 'bum' is not an option.

The pub was under new management, so I stumbled over and asked James, the manager, if any bar jobs were available. That afternoon, three pints of cider down, I was in the office interviewing my drunk little heart out. Score ... I had the job!

Although no bar positions were available, he was recruiting a chef. I know, it sounds like a far stretch, but I did have some skills in the kitchen. At the time, my mum was a restaurateur, so I had seen how a commercial kitchen worked. Plus, the student bar didn't have a Michelin menu – a working knowledge of a deep-fat fryer and a microwave would do!

When I heard the words, 'You've got the job,' it felt like a small but significant victory. I was so happy and proud of myself, I ordered my fourth pint. I then fell off my bar stool. Perhaps the floor was a little uneven – it couldn't have possibly been my inebriation. My new boss, James, laughed it off. Was this a good sign?

LIKING A BAD BOY IS NOT A GOOD THING

Working in pubs is great if you don't want to be seen. Everyone is drunk, the music is loud, the lights are dimly lit, and the busyness means no one has time for deep conversations. Perfect! I was working hard and playing harder. I would pull off a string of AFDs (all fucking day) shifts. We would start at 10 a.m., set up shop, clear down at 11 p.m., and drink until closing time.

My hard graft paid off. While my duties were limited to the kitchen, it wasn't long before my outgoing demeanour and ability to work around the clock without complaining was clocked by James. I was moved on to tills and soon I was working from 10 a.m. until 2 a.m. – slipping into an exhaustive pattern of working and drinking, with one hour of sleep a night.

When you are spending every day in one pub, the locals become your friends and your friends become your family. I don't know if I should say this, but it was so much fun. The camaraderie was infectious; the music was blasting, the bar was four deep with thirsty punters and I was in my element of extremism.

And let's not forget the sex. It was incredibly easy to find the sex. In fact, at one point, I was deliberating over three different men and wondering who I would date first. As I mentioned earlier, it's a fairly common trait of those with MRKH to be promiscuous. It's got nothing to do with sex, though. It's validation.

The more sex I had, the more I earned my place in womanhood.

For a while, I only slept with 'punters' who came into the pub for a drink, but then it moved closer to home. Attracting the wandering eye of my manager boosted my non-existent ego. It started off with the odd flirt here and there, a bottle of WKD Blue and a cigarette. Then it was a drunken fumble in the pub across the road ... and then it was a full-blown fling. We were having sex on the office floor after the pub closed. We were being caught by other staff members. Sometimes, we would splash out on cheap hotels.

After a number of months, we went from secret lovers to an exclusive couple with our entire lives ahead of us.

In the excitement of our romance, I didn't stop to tell him about my MRKH diagnosis. I didn't want to; I was in denial and didn't think I needed to; I would do it one day in the future. Unfortunately, my secret got out before I had a chance to share it.

After I had an argument with a co-worker one night, she decided to tell my boyfriend that his girlfriend had no womb and was born without a vagina. She announced this, very loudly, during a quiet afternoon shift in the bar in front of a roomful of regulars. James didn't look amused; however, the locals did.

As everyone stared at me – the bartender born with no vagina – James pointed at me and said, 'Is it any wonder I don't want to have sex with THAT?'

I thought his sex drive was low. I didn't think it was me.

CHAPTER 6

What do you deserve?

Amazingly, James and I didn't break up after that night. We didn't, however, ever speak of my diagnosis again. Gradually, I sloped away from living at home with Mum, and moved in with James and his flatmate. It made sense at the time. They lived five minutes from the pub, and I was unable to look my mum in the eye anymore. The shame was too much. She knew I was imploding and taking life to a dangerous edge. She knew I was desperate, and I wasn't going to allow her to see me like this.

I would never let her know what came next.

Being extremely drunk or disgustingly hungover will cause irrational behaviour. I know, I am stating the obvious. James and I lived our life to the extreme: extreme tiredness, extreme highs and lows, extreme alcohol abuse, extreme spending and extreme emotional outbursts.

I can't remember the first time James hit me.

I can't remember feeling like I should leave him. I can't remember my reasons for staying. I can't remember how I justified it all at the time. I remember hitting him back – not just that first time, but on various occasions afterwards. It became how we argued: we would get drunk, laugh and fight.

We had a reputation as a turbulent, 'passionate' couple. While people saw our snide remarks and sheer venom for one another, they never saw the fighting. On the rare occasions I did speak up, I muttered how we should not be together, but I never left. We were addicted to this mutual destruction.

Since then, I've read more – and tried to understand – the idea of a 'mutually abusive' relationship. Mutually abusive is a concept used when describing a relationship where both partners are abusive to each other. According to some experts, it's a myth and there is always one partner with a balance of power. Was it self-defence; was I the survivor or another abuser? These are the questions I continue to ask myself, and I'm not sure I'll ever find an answer.

I know this part of my story is going to cause a divide. No man should ever strike a woman, but no woman should strike a man. We fought as a couple. In the depths of our drunken splurges and bender comedowns, I would spit rage. I would force him to climb down our apartment building as he had no other way of escaping me. I would pour cleaning chemicals in the bath when he was trying to wash. I was not blameless; I am not blameless.

This relationship was the product of two people who didn't have the know-how, maturity, clarity, self-worth or compassion to let each other go. This was a co-dependent relationship between two people who were in the thick of their sickness. Hurt people hurt people. Sick people make sick choices.

I would stand in the shower, holding the side of my waist, after being karate-kicked in the ribs. I would stand in the shower, clutching my ear, after being smacked so hard all I could hear was ringing. I would lie on the floor in the back room of the pub, when no one else was there, after he hit me to the ground. I would sit on the bathroom floor and allow his fury to urinate on me, literally.

We were both in denial, hiding from the truth of what we were living in. One night, on a random crusade, we went on a mission to rescue my friend who was in a physically abusive relationship. It didn't hit home that I wasn't rescuing myself.

We were sick, damaged, and I despised him. I despised his ability to find himself in financial debt, for taking drugs, for introducing me to drugs and for hurting me.

When your self-esteem is so low, it can feel like you have nowhere to go. I felt like I owed any man gratitude for 'taking me on'. I felt like I should be grateful to any man for sticking with me after learning my truth. If violence was the by-product of that, so be it.

This is a hard chapter to write because I know how it sounds. Today, I would be the first to advocate for women (and men) to leave a domestic-violence situation. Back then, however, that was my reality. Plus, after years of physically harming myself, this was a 'known' feeling. It came with a strange sense of belonging.

PRAYING FOR A MISTAKE

Sometimes, I would buy a pregnancy test. I knew I could never get pregnant naturally, but I wanted to feel the experience of peeing on a stick. I wanted to know what it felt like waiting for the 'positive' lines to appear.

I also wanted to believe that the doctors had made a mistake – that I could carry a baby all along and my body had the pieces they believed were missing. I wanted to feel like other women felt – to experience joyful anticipation, hope and elation as I told my partner, 'We are having a baby.'

Isn't a pregnancy stick the only measuring stick to being a woman? If I can't do that, what use am I to anyone?

As a self-confessed emotional risk-taker, I was still adamant to see how far I could push my limits. On a rare evening off from working behind the bar, I, James and a group of people sat in front of the bar, boozing the night away.

Drunk and sad, I thought about what life would look like if, for just one second, there was a way out. Another way to earn money. Another place I could belong. Another way to self-sabotage. Another escape route.

I had always idolised the idea of living in London – a city only a couple of hours from Reading, which seemed to hold so many possibilities. Of course, I could have moved to London and got a bar job with my experience, but that was far too logical for my scattered, destructive mindset.

Instead, I turned to a stranger who was drinking beside me and asked, 'Do you know the name of any pimps in London who might be looking for working girls?'

I was extremely drunk but deadly serious. I had heard about sex workers making a good living in cities and it didn't feel such a far stretch from my current life – using my body as a product, not a part of me.

To my surprise, he had a name and a phone number (just my bad luck!). Before I knew it, I was in a taxi to London. I hadn't told James or my friends that I was leaving the pub. I just walked out and nobody even noticed. Scary, really, how your absence is so easily forgotten.

From the back of the taxi, I called this mysterious pimp, who told me about a location in London where I would be met. I could sleep there and also work from there. It was strangely and surreally easy to set up my new life as a sex worker, even in a country where sex work is illegal.

I must have passed out in the taxi, as I vaguely remember the driver pulling into a service station to fill the tank up with petrol. When the bright lights of the petrol station woke me up, what I was doing suddenly hit home – and I realised I did not want to be there.

'Turn around,' I told the driver, 'I need to get back to Reading.'

An hour later, he was pulling back up at the pub that I'd left. I worked my way through the crowds; back to my drink, James and my friends. No one asked where I'd gone and I never told them.

SEARCHING FOR SAFETY

My relationship with James went on for five more years – a crazy amount of time when I look back now.

After James got reposted to another pub with the same company, I eventually followed him up to Leicester. My loyalty landed me an assistant manager role at a pub a few miles away from James's new place of work. I hoped this was the beginning of a new life, but, in reality, it was just another geographical sidestep. I was changing my landscape, but not my life.

We had a lovely little flat in the centre of Leicester. For a while it did get better. Leaving the past behind felt cleansing. We decorated and ate fancy high-end takeaway meals on our day off. My manager was a good friend of James's, who valued my work and, eventually, some sense of pride was being restored for the both of us.

What I know now, I didn't know then. If abuse takes place in a relationship, unless a structured and therapeutic treatment plan is applied, bursts of happiness are nothing but dangerous bandages. On most occasions, the healthiest, safest and kindest act this couple can do is to walk away from each other.

After a year working as an assistant manager, I applied for a licensed house manager position in James's sister pub. It was a converted barge that had a retractable roof. I thought, 'Maybe, Ally, this will fix everything.'

Of course, I was on the move again, with no plan to look inward.

At this point, James and I were complete strangers sharing a bed. We both had wandering eyes, and it wasn't long before we both realised that our attention was no longer for each other. There was no big 'happening' that finally paved the way for an event.

After everything we had been through, it was James who acknowledged that the abuse had to stop. That we were not a couple in love, but a couple in the depths of not knowing any other way. Until he did. The debt, the drugs, the alcohol, the fighting – it was incessant.

I remember clinging to 'us' right until the end. Even at this well-overdue realisation that we shouldn't be together, I stood on the steps of his pub, begging him to reverse his decision to end things. Begging.

I still wasn't prepared to leave. This is a pattern of mine, which even now I have to be aware of, whether it's an unhealthy relationship, job or any kind of commitment. Twisting, torquing and rinsing every last bit of blood out of a relationship, because I didn't know my worth. I didn't want to regret and lose love.

Was this ever love in the first place?

Today, I don't dislike James, wherever he is. I hope he found some healing and, of course, I hope he hasn't continued his abusive patterns. I am not angry and I do not feel like a victim. An important part of my story and my healing is taking responsibility for my share of our relationship.

Depression has this way of dressing itself up as a bad day or a broken heart. But depression is so much more than that. At times, we find ourselves negotiating with depression and deny its role in our lives. When we see someone else's silent struggle or abuse, our instincts kick in to help them. But when it's our own depressive state, we turn and look the other way, in fear that if we don't, it may win.

When James finally ended it (because this wasn't our first go at a breakup), I really knew (and accepted) it was over.

I got in a taxi at 1 a.m. and asked to go 'home'. I walked up my mum's pathway, knocked on the door and burst into tears. I was exhausted from travelling across the country and I was exhausted from feeling like I didn't deserve to be loved or to love myself.

For a long time, I hid this chapter of my story, or I downplayed it. I didn't acknowledge the extremes of the abuse, even to myself – the times when my face was so bruised that I didn't recognise my own reflection.

Looking back at my younger self, the one with the bloodshot eyes and bruises, I would tell her that it doesn't need to be that way. I would praise and applaud her bravery. I would give her permission to cry. None of us can change a person who isn't ready to change. We need to accept that a person may need to sit at rock bottom, before seeing a way out. For all those young girls and women who justify sadness because they feel they deserve it, I'm sorry, but you are wrong.

What you are, in fact, is beautiful, courageous, whole and complete.

You are enough. You are so enough that one day, you'll be too much. Too much for the wrong person, the pain and heartache. Your 'enoughness' is going to create opportunities and the best love stories ever; better than the ones in the movies.

Your enoughness has always been there. I just hope it doesn't take too long, and too much grief, to find it. When you do, I will be cheerleading you from the stands and shouting, 'Welcome home to healing!'

CHAPTER 7

I was tired of being a passenger in life

After fleeing James in the middle of the night, I begged my mum to help me. She called my area manager at the bar and explained that I was 200 miles away from work. I was too tired, ashamed and embarrassed to call myself, and uncertain if I had a life to return to in Leicester. James had called my mum to see if I was OK, but that was it.

At Mum's, I spent most of my time nibbling on toast, sleeping, crying and trying to understand what the hell was going on. I still felt like a child trying to cope in an adult's world. Funnily enough, a pattern was starting to emerge. A pattern that, today, is making perfect sense. I was an 'emotional sprinter' – when my emotions are heightened, my instinct is to go. Somewhere, anywhere.

When a fight happened, I ran to the pub. When trauma hit, I ran to Australia. When abuse happened, I ran home. When reality hit me, I ran to self-harm. I never knew how to stay, resolve and remain in discomfort. So many of us don't, especially when there are so many escapes at our fingertips. Social media. Alcohol. A plane ticket. A job resignation.

It goes back to the geography thing – when the going gets tough, we get going. If I change my address, I will change my feelings. If

I change my hair, I will change my worth. If I change my job, I will change my aspirations. Sometimes, change is the last thing any of us want, despite thinking it will save us.

Why are we so wired to crave change, but feel so damn uncomfortable when we get it?

Today, I do everything I can to fight this urge. If I am in chaos, I stay ridiculously still. I never make a decision from a place of immense euphoria or devastating loss. My motto is: when you don't know what to do, avoid doing anything at all. The less mapwork involved, the more self-work can evolve.

Put the suitcase away, stay, and see that being a passenger on any trip is a *pretty* powerless place to live.

It took me a long time to get to this point, of course. There would be many more moves after James – some that took me back and some that brought me forward. When I returned to Reading after my break-up, what my parents didn't know was that I had already started reapplying for jobs ... back in Leicester.

I didn't want to go back to James. I didn't want to go back to that life, but I also felt the urge to sprint from my current stage – and my current location.

How many of us do that, right?

We exhaust our resilience to the point where we have no energy to leave, even if we could. The back-and-forth process to any break-up is wrought with fear. We debate with our grief. Will I ever love someone again? Will I be loved? Will I find a soulmate? Will I find a sex-mate? We don't want to leave a bad relationship because we fear what is on the other side of sadness.

When you have been beaten down, both emotionally and physically, and don't know how to be alone, it's easy to slip into 'maybe I am better off here'.

Wrong. I get it, I've felt it. Your mind is playing tricks on you.

I urge you never, ever to stay in a relationship that is hurting you. That is not love, it's routine. It's not true love, it's guilt and regret. Think back to when you were a kid daydreaming about what life as a 'grown-up' would look like. Did it look like plates smashing, name-calling, hand-raising and manipulation? I am going to say, no? Because for me, it didn't. For me, I only saw simple but incredible love.

I wasn't capable of love; not for me, not for a partner, and certainly not for James and me as a couple.

I did, however, want to feel safe. Only then, I knew it as control.

So, less than two months after my break-up with James, I fell in love again – a different kind of love, not violent but just as complex and confusing. A love that began as a long-distance relationship but then became my escape route. Again. Another way to leave behind my past and try to reclaim my future.

I was still living at my mum's house when I announced to my parents that I was in love with Tom – a bartender from the pub I used to work for in Loughborough. We had been dating for over a year at this point, visiting each other on weekends and sending thousands of text messages in between.

If you know the pub industry, you know that it can be quite, hmmm, 'close'. Due to long hours, late nights and days off drinking in the very same pub, everyone knows everyone. When one pub gets boring, you go to the next. I met Tom because he worked for James, my ex.

I get it, I was literally shitting on my doorstep. It was like that. Tom was quirky, like me, and he was fiercely protective over my dysfunctional relationship with James. He would always text me to see if I was OK after an argument. He was a friend, but I knew I wanted more. Being the serial dater I was, staying single after James was *not* an option.

Now, as I explained to my mum, I wanted to go 'all in' and move in with him. So I packed a suitcase (again), got on a train (again) and prepared to start a new chapter (again!).

When I arrived back in the Midlands it was midday, and Tom was asleep from a late-night barshift. It was not the big welcome I was hoping for. In fact, it was scarily lonely and underwhelming. But me being me, I tip-toed quietly around our Loughborough rental house, and poured myself a drink to settle in. I had landed a role with a hotel chain as an assistant manager – a job that would see me living half the week in the hotel.

I hated it. I was tired and felt so out of place. I didn't have the finesse required for a hotel lobby and I was becoming more and more vacant as a woman. I respected that Tom worked hard, and that his job, with the same company I jumped ship from, was flourishing. I didn't feel like 'Queen Bee' as his girlfriend, but a woman home alone on a Friday night, chain-smoking and thinking, 'Why am I here?'

I did love Tom. He was funny and kooky. He was odd in all the right ways and he wanted to be with me. We rarely discussed a future with children (erm, ideal), and we loved the idea of saving money hard. Our passion for travel was big, and we were young enough to never fear having a planless-plan.

It really wasn't Tom's fault that I was too broken to be there. I didn't applaud his 100-hour work week, but neither did I challenge it. I just drank more, stayed out late, found people who would love me, and wobbled home in time for curfew. He wasn't my parent, but nor could he be a loving boyfriend, because I didn't know how to be in love.

We never discussed my diagnosis. It never came up, because I never let it.

AND SHE'S OFF AGAIN

The hotel industry wasn't for me. It was a clumsily run business. After growing up in my mum's restaurant and climbing the pub ladder fast, I knew business and standards. This particular employer didn't meet the standards. So, I quit. All this moving and shifting was giving me confidence in my skills as a survivor. I was starting to realise, I would always be able to find work — even if the work wasn't a daydream vocation.

After door-to-door knocking around local agencies, I landed a job in a call centre. Every day, I would negotiate with irate customers who had fallen victim to cash redemption claims as part of a big mobile phone company. It was actually quite effortless. I was working steady hours, surrounded by a bunch of misfits like me; unsure of what their life-plan should be.

But I was so ... confused. I knew deep down inside was a person who loved creativity and hard work. It was almost like watching myself in a movie, where I was shouting at the screen, only to find the leading lady couldn't hear me. I was drifting from one fucked-up choice to the next. I was alone at night, and in the call centre by day.

Tom and I would spend the occasional morning together, but mostly we would argue. We would argue about him not being home enough, and my gripes that he couldn't comfort me enough. I would find my way into late-night binges, strangers' homes and friendships that weren't simple. I was repeating the past, but with more expertise on how to make it harder. See, I wanted hard. I wanted to be challenged; the only problem was, I didn't know how.

Typically, most teenagers will grow out of self-harming. Much like an eating disorder, there can be a shelf-life. At 26 years old, I was still hurting myself; admittedly less, but the tendencies were there. A colleague of mine at the hotel once said, 'Ally, aren't you embarrassed to wear sleeves that show your arms?' Up until this point, I wasn't. I would never wear super-revealing clothes, but I never realised if, on the odd occasion, I was bringing the hotel shame. As someone born into compassion, even when I hated every inch of my body, I also knew that I wasn't doing it because I was bored. I was hurting myself because I was bereft.

I was hoping for openness, and not a shutdown from my colleague. So what did I do? I put on my favourite track of the time, 'I Believe', by Blessid Union of Souls (shit, I believe again!), and hurt myself. I chose a different way this time. A way I had not explored before. I don't know why – maybe because I didn't feel anything differently. That was the last time I self-harmed, not because it was so painful, but because it was on a body part that I knew was too hard to explain away. It had to be the last time, because I was out of excuses.

The last time I blamed it on an oil burn from a deep-fat fryer. It wasn't. I have always claimed it was, until this day. It was easier that way.

Unfortunately, a different way means a different healing method, one which I didn't know how to do. The scar didn't heal, it grew. So much that my friend took me to get it medically treated. I wasn't in much pain, but the shame was so intense. The bandage was peeking from under my top, where Tom asked me what happened. He knew I was spiralling.

A month later, we were on a plane to Australia. I was on the run again.

AUSTRALIA, ROUND TWO

As soon as I stepped onto the Melburnian tarmac, I wondered if my life would look like the hit series *Home and Away*, despite being 545 miles south of the famous 'Summer Bay'.

With impressive hospitality experience, Tom and I landed a job running a restaurant in the amazing Apollo Bay.

On our first night there, we drank a 'VB', otherwise known as 'Victorian Bitter', a no-go beer for Aussie locals. I was on a mission to make this work – this being my reincarnation as an Australian. Because of my mum's heritage, I could get an Australian passport, which meant I could stay ... for good.

With a desire to make my mum proud, Tom and I worked hard, saved harder and attempted to make a new life in the sun. The only problem was, Melbourne had more rain than sun – not the beachy lifestyle I imagined. Undeterred, we went out partying and drinking, sparked up our sex life and decided that, maybe, this was going to be the future that helped us find 'our love'.

Sure, it was fun. We had a great laugh, and saved good money, but with bosses on acid and an owner asleep, we knew that this job needed to wrap itself up. Off to the Big 'Sydney' Apple we went to find new work and, hopefully, finally settle.

Tom got a job in recruitment, and I got a job working in IT support. There is one thing you should know about me. I am a mess when it comes to maths, IT and anything technical. I can muscle through YouTube, but working full time for a major Australian corporate brand was going to be a stretch, even for me.

Tom said to me, 'Think of happiness like a pair of scales. Do you want happiness or money? Money or happiness?' I had never had money, and I didn't know happiness, so for six months I would be the girl who would confidently say, 'Have you tried turning the printer on and off again?' For the most part, that advice worked.

It wasn't too long before we were living in what felt like a treehouse, overlooking the beautiful Bondi Beach. We would see the possums on our terracotta balcony, the kookaburras at brekkie, and hear the rolling surf faintly in the background. It was heaven. I felt like I was living out my mother's attempt at happiness. I felt like I was honouring her past, while redesigning my future.

Sure, I could work in the corporate slog, wear fancy clothes and look the part – I was the actress being all successful. And we were making good money. I would always take care of the finances. It was like a fun game. Thousand here, thousand there and a thousand to play around with. It was incredible.

Looking back on it now, we were not trying to fulfil the 'Bondi Bubble' stereotype. Yes, we were well-earning Brits, but Bondi is a mecca for more than that. Bondi Beach has this magnetism about it that attracts hopefuls. This iconic suburb is a place that welcomes the 'black sheep of the family', those with big dreams on little budgets, and those who haven't found their 'home' yet.

For me, home was and still is wherever my family lives – England. But I mean a different type of home.

I would look at the ocean from the bus stop on my way to work and the taxi window as I left my office. Unlike Melbourne, where we'd spend our evenings in bars, rarely did Tom and I go out in Bondi. We also never went to the beach for the first six years that we lived there. He didn't love crowds or sand or swimming. At that point, I didn't realise that my greatest love to come was the ocean.

I was living in someone else's version of a dream. Families save for years for what was my backyard. I was living in heaven.

The only thing that was missing was me.

THE UNDOING OF A 'SAFE' RELATIONSHIP

My version of the word safe has changed a lot – you will understand later in my story why. Back then, safe meant sturdy. A sturdy income, a sturdy rental agreement and even a sturdy weekly meal plan.

On a Saturday, instead of basking at the water's edge, we would wander up to Bondi Junction (otherwise known as Bondi Junkyard) to do our weekly grocery shop. Tom would baste my pale body in SPF 50 sun lotion. While I believe in being sun-smart, I couldn't understand why I was being treated like an ill-informed child – the first sign of real cracks in our relationship.

I knew what the sun did. I knew that, to get sunburnt, you needed sun. But we were in a shopping mall. When we weren't, we were watching reruns of British sitcoms. I was living in Australia, but I was living in Britain ... and I never really understood why.

It wasn't all bad, especially compared to my previous violent relationship. This was loving, respectful and had a lot of kindness. At first, our sex life was good (I always orgasmed with Tom!). Our childlessness meant that we had more money than most. We had freedom and the means to explore it.

Although we didn't go out in our town, we did travel further afield. We were living in Australia where we had instant access to Fiji, Bali and the beautiful tropics in Queensland. Our bank balance meant we could afford private villas, beaches and high-end resorts. We would sip champagne, order top-notch steaks, and never blinked at buying a first-class flight ticket.

In terms of financial success, I had made it. From the outside, we were a soaring, successful couple. I was the envy of friends back home who were ridden with motherhood. I was the person who had left destruction for a life down under.

If you saw me, you'd think I had it all. So, why did the thought of stepping onto the beach terrify me? And why didn't my partner ever question it?

I DELETED MY VAGINA POST

I find ambition super-sexy. While it keeps me on my successful toes, seeing a man driven is attractive and contagious. My parents both demonstrated the importance of finding your way, and although I don't seek out power, if a man had a splash of it, I was in!

With a successful career building in international recruitment, Tom found himself travelling interstate often. With that, I discovered a new freedom.

I was alone a lot – and I loved it. I was finally living in the freedom that allowed me to be me.

With every night he was away, I found myself scrolling through Facebook trying to find women like me. I would search the word 'vaginaless' hoping to find women that felt the emptiness and displacement that I did. Did they have a vagina? Did they feel like women? Did they rattle their boobs trying to find their own version of womanhood like me?

One night, I found myself pouring my heart out to strangers online. I had logged on to a forum for women with MRKH, telling the entire online space that I had been born without a vagina and a womb, and the words just kept flowing. Maybe the emotions took over or maybe the attention did. At that moment, I realised, I was writing for the first time freely. I was telling my truth.

'I am Ally, and I was born without a vagina. Ally, who was born without a cervix. Ally, who was born without a womb.'

Fuck.

I wrote my post, 'Becoming Ally', thinking it would never be read, but really, the person I feared would read it first was in fact Tom. I needed to unleash this secret that I had been carrying for years. It was killing me from the soul outwards. So, I deleted the post. Months later, I would share it again, and save it, this time.

Yet in so many ways, I knew that Tom wouldn't recognise the person that I wanted to become. I wasn't going to be the 'Ally' anymore that he met all those years before on a bar stool.

The thing is, it was never his fault that I was living constantly on the sidelines of life.

That's the thing about a rocky relationship; everyone plays their part. Their undoing? Being unfeeling, and certainly unloving.

CHAPTER 8

When the break-up needs to happen

The last thing I ever want to be seen as is a victim. Not that I don't believe victims need to have their safe place, voice and rescue, because so many do. For me, the term victim transports me back to what hurt me and leaves me unable to heal. In some circumstances, I was a victim of physical or emotional abuse. However, I had to make a very conscious decision to rid the residue of a toxic time. More importantly, I had to take a long and hard look at my role in someone else's pain.

Because I *did* cause pain. I was exasperating, confused, erratic and unsafe. Sometimes I would go for a drink after work with colleagues, go silent on Tom, and not go home for two days. I would roll into my corporate Sydney gig, wearing the clothes from the night before, looking remorseful and dishevelled. I was secretive about my friends and guarded my mobile phone as well as I could. Sometimes, I didn't guard my phone well enough and Tom would start asking questions: 'Why are you getting messages from random men in the early hours of the morning?' 'Why did you pay $80 for a taxi when you said you were working?'

My excuses would never quite appease the man who wanted to love me and leave me all at once.

It's funny writing a memoir, because while I want to impress and inspire you, I can't bullshit you. I can't give you a story that portrays me as a woman suffering in the grips of a misused body. I was also cruel, thoughtless and just as powerful with how I inflicted pain. There are no excuses to abuse any person, not just a woman.

While we are championing the equal rights of vulnerable women, I once threw a cup of boiling water across a room, narrowly missing Tom. I would scream at him in the early hours of the morning, picking arguments with no foundations. The next day, my neighbours would stare back at me with disgust. So many days, I would talk about why we shouldn't be together and then beg him to stay when he agreed.

I was a mess and I knew that it was finally time to wake up to the hangovers, broken plates, alienated neighbours ... and shame.

While it's not easy, or even possible, for everyone to lay the past to an amicable rest, I have spent the last ten years holding conversations with those who hurt me – and whom I hurt too. If we have the ability to reconnect with the people who became part of our darkest chapters, then we have a chance at mending what broke us. We have the gift of apologising, resolving and unravelling the facts, to understand the lessons. It's not always a movie-scene apology, sometimes it's quieter or weirder than that.

I cannot write this story if I don't fess up to my behaviour either. At some point, blame must rest with us too, if we have a chance of awakening to our lost selves. I shouldn't say 'blame', because that's just another title we don't need. Perhaps the better way of saying it is that we need to take ownership of any relationship ending. We all have questions, fears, guilt-stricken moments and rock bottoms. But it is so important to acknowledge:

Provocation doesn't equal abuse-justification.

Excuses don't make it OK (or better).

When to take accountability and when to label it abuse.

No story is ever the same, but the messages ring clear: a break-up is a series of events that can be unequal, untold and, sometimes, incorrectly forgiven. It's easy to have wisdom ten years *after* a messy break-up. It might even take a series of brutal break-ups to see that love had left long before the end. It's all about trust. Trusting that this person was meant for you, even to teach a yucky lesson. Trusting that the insights will one day come. Trusting that you won't make the same mistake twice.

For the second time, I found myself not ending a relationship that should have ended. For all the moments I hurled verbal abuse, caused distrust and denied Tom the truth about my past, I am truly sorry. He was, and is, a good man. And good things deserve to happen to good people. I truly hope this is the case for Tom now.

WHEN YOU KNOW, YOU KNOW

As my relationship with Tom broke down, my familial relationships grew stronger. Every night when Tom was at work, I would chat to my mum on the phone for hours. We were having the conversations that had been absent for the last ten years.

We would cry and shiver at the honesty being shared. It felt like a reunion with my mum. It felt like the 'trauma ice' was being broken. It was all because I was learning who I was, outside of the controlling relationship that sadly Tom's and mine was.

I would start to drip-feed truth bombs about the times when I fucked up or stayed out all night. I would selectively explain my new-found insights, which of course my red-wine head amped up. Despite knowing I was in a relationship that should have ended five years in (and which was now sitting at nine), I would share how much money we were earning, and the next tropical holiday we'd booked. I was faking freedom.

Every Saturday, while the droves of tourists would head for the beach, sun-kissed and jacked up on vitamin D, Tom and I would walk to Coles supermarket (again!). We did this every Saturday. With him hating the sun, and me unwilling to break the cycle of rigid routines, I would walk beside him, sometimes behind.

As the ocean was becoming smaller in the distance, and the concrete ugliness of Bondi Junction got bigger, I would bargain with my must-haves. On repeat I would say:

Ally, so what if you only have sex once a year for the rest of your life? You go on great holidays.
Ally, so what if you have no friends? You have Tom.
Ally, so what if you are working in a job that gives you no joy? You earn great money.
Ally, so what if you miss your parents? They don't have to see this.
Ally, so what if you are unhappy most of the time? At least you are safe.

Can I just clear my throat for a moment and say, 'Ahem, the word safety in this context is utter bullshit.'

I absolutely, categorically and certainly, was not living in my version of safety. Sure, I was safer from the world I created in Liverpool where I couldn't remember the night before. I was safer from one-night stands in back alleys and deserted parks. I was safer from self-harm because the Australian climate doesn't lend itself to wearing long sleeves every day. And in many ways, I was safe because I was letting someone else decide my life for me.

Here is when the blame game rears its head. If we choose to conform to something we know is wrong, are we emotionally abused, or complicit? I wanted to be in an environment with someone who loved me, so that they would protect me from myself. But at some point, the lines become blurred between being supportive and being summoned.

I gave Tom every reason to be cautious with me anytime I said I wanted to go for a post-drink tipple. These are the same people who would be my playmates for a three-day bender. I didn't have any other friends in Australia. I remember thinking, if Tom goes away and something happens to me, I don't have anyone to call for help. I have no friends, no family and no 'emergency contact'. I was so alone it was scary.

At some point – driven by guilt, I'm sure – I decided to play a new role: the over-doting 'wife'.

It was similar to the days when I would take a pregnancy test just to show I could play the role of a woman. If I couldn't be a mother, I could be the good wife. Every day, I would make sure Tom's keys, bus pass and wallet were neatly stacked on the table. Every morning, I would choose his clothes and lay them out in the bedroom next door. In the winter, I would warm the clothes on a heater, while Tom took a shower. When I did start going to Bondi Icebergs in the summer, one of Sydney's most iconic beachside hangouts, I would go early enough that I would be home in time for his first cup of tea.

The thing is, I did love him. Hugely. He was funny, intelligent, a little weird but kind. He helped me with IT and bank stuff, and would spoon me at night. He was my best friend, and the two of us didn't know how to end things, because really, for him too, familiarity was better than change. He was safe in my support and financial planning. We all have reasons for finding a routine that isn't right for our souls, but it can be right for our hearts, even when it's so wrong for our lives.

A MOTHER'S BACKSTORY CAN SAVE YOU TOO

A therapist once said to me that I idolise my mum. Even thinking about this statement now, I still feel a little grumpy and insulted, with her labelling my mum as my hero. Like, I couldn't be my own idol and create my own life-moving content. She inferred that I was clutching at the inspirational stories of others. Isn't it possible that respect can be mistaken for imitation? Is it possible that unconditional love can be mistaken for copy-catting a parent?

Either way, she was bloody brave, and I love her every day for it.

I do get it. My mum and I are insanely similar. We say the same things at the exact same time. We hold hands when talking, laugh at our crudeness and have no problem with talking about the sticky stuff in life. We both wear hair in top-buns, live in jeans and share what I can only say is a magical bond. I was picked out for her, and she was selected for me. It was a partnership destined before I was even conceived.

There is also the harder stuff too, which could be construed as learnt behaviour. My mum suffered from anorexia, self-harmed and found herself walking the streets of Sydney with no concept of home. I too had given eating disorders a good go, self-harmed my way through my twenties, and found myself, 30 years later, strolling the same streets.

Mum's family were disjointed, broken and silenced by society's politeness not to expose a broken family. It simply was not the 'done' thing back then.

My grandmother Mary (Mum's mum) was also a woman who struggled with life. After being abandoned by her husband (my grandfather), she fell into a destructive addiction to painkillers. While Mum and her sister were at school, Mary was at home in bed catatonic, drugged up to the eyeballs and grieving her lost marriage. On the weekends, my mum would clean the house, while Mary would lie in dirty bed sheets and squalor. On weekdays, Mary would work, but then go home, closing her bedroom door behind her.

Nowadays, my mum and her sister would have been taken into care. But back then, you didn't dare talk about a broken marriage, an addicted and mentally unwell mother, and a father who disappeared with another woman. Once, my mum explained to me that Mary chased her around the house with a kitchen knife. On another occasion, Mary called the police, reporting that my mum had been a victim of rape. But no such act of rape had occurred. While this statement by Mary was based off a drug-induced paranoia, the unspeakable to come actually *did* happen.

As a former Eastern Suburbs girl, I knew the apartment block that mum had lived in. The same apartment she was actually nearly raped in, by an intruder who was never caught by the police. After he broke through an open window, my mum knew what she had to do to survive. After reading a book about a prostitute 'talking men out of rape', Mum attempted to do the same. She talked to him for hours, naked, with a gun held to her head. And he never did rape her. Her ability to personalise with her attacker saved her life.

Even her anorexia and self-harm were not treated professionally, because eating disorders and mental health were better hidden than heard about back then. She was left to fend for herself, fight her own battles and learn what motherless love felt like.

I mean, really, what had she lived through?
What had become her own version of 'normal'?
How brave does one woman have to be, before help is offered?

I am not sharing these stories because my mum's backstory deserves to be told with a punchy strapline. In fact, it startles me how she never really spoke to anyone about it. She doesn't do praise, acknowledgement or public speeches.

I feel that her bravery deserves to be told. I want to do the one thing that so many denied her, and that's giving her a voice worth hearing. And because it was her past that was going to alter my future.

We were and are different. All of our stories are. You can't repeat or duplicate our pasts, despite all of us wanting to fit into a box, category or drop-down menu. The difference between my mum and I was that I knew love awaited me. It was just that back then, I wasn't ready to feel the love, because I was too ashamed to accept it.

So maybe, yeah, I do idolise her. I was also deeply grateful when we could share our truths with each other – when we both saw each other as flawed but worthy humans.

If she could overcome bravery, so could I. It is Mum's love, scars and past pains that allow me to share as in-depth as I do. We always will, and this is a love that I have never been uncertain of.

Just like my dad, whose love wanted to save me too.

WHEN LYING BECOMES TOO TIRING

My mum, being Australian, would come over for a couple of months a year to visit me and Tom. In our first ten years in Australia, we would travel back to England frequently. Tom would have preferred less, but for me, it was a non-negotiable. I always knew the day I couldn't travel 'home' was the day I didn't want to be in Australia anymore.

So, we compromised. My holidays back to the UK were pretty much about me flaunting an enviable lifestyle. I was the girl living in Bondi Beach. I was based in one of the most desirable cities in the world, alongside oceans and exotic islands. From the outside I was winning, and my social status was making up for everything I was lacking.

Lacking happiness and fertility, and having a vagina that I wasn't at peace with. Inside, I was screaming. I was still reasoning with my previous escapes; nights of promiscuity, hedonism and cup throwing.

My life back in Bondi was a postcard of success, but I wasn't living. I was existing.

In my eyes, back then, if you lived this close to unliving, there was no risk of it going wrong.

If you walked quietly, refrained from friendships, avoided busy beaches and went back home for just 15 days a year, then there was no risk of fucking up again.

For those of us who out-expire a break-up, we blame or hate ourselves for not leaving earlier. We tell ourselves off for not being strong or brave enough to leave at the first signs of a red flag. Our friends or close colleagues will blatantly ask us, 'Why are you still with him?' Like it's just easy to walk away.

But like giving up something you love that's bad for you, there is never the 'right' time to leave a relationship. Sometimes a departure is interrupted by a health scare, financial fall-out or a loss in the family. Before we know it, we are negotiating once again with our happiness. We will tell our deflated selves, 'I will just wait until ... I will just see if ... I want to make sure that ...'

We are simply not wired to plan for heartbreak. It's better to know what we can see than to plan for a life we can't. Despite daydreaming about a life that could be so incredible, we settle for a life that is guaranteed: set mealtimes, monthly budgets, Instagram perfection, trending audios and a postcard existence.

Until it's not.

WHEN YOUR PARTNER BECOMES A STRANGER

One night when I got home from work, instead of putting on my baggy no-elastic PJs, I put a sheer camisole tee-thingy. Tom and I were in a sexless relationship at this stage and had been for five of the ten years we'd been together. The only time we would have sex was on my birthday, which, in Australia, fell on a public holiday. This meant, while in Australia, I would never have to work on my birthday. Taking advantage of this extra day off, we would always go away somewhere super-pretty and super-expensive. We fed our feelings with money. Wrapped up in balmy nights and birthday cocktails, it made sense that this was our yearly 'sex day'.

Outside of that, nothing. So, it made no sense that when at home, I would try to woo him. Maybe I was desperate. Maybe I was trying to rekindle a lost flame. But maybe I was petrified that our relationship was uncoiling at a rapid rate, and I would do anything and everything to save it.

Don't forget, I am Ally, the girl who refuses to give up and is never the 'dumper', but the 'dumpee'.

Everything was so odd.

We were acting super-polite to one another. The kind of politeness you give someone you've never liked, but you know pain is coming for them. We would talk about the future as single people. We never ate together. We didn't even argue anymore. We both were contemplating what sex with other people would be like. More importantly, we were both contemplating what *loving* with other people would be like.

Later that week, calmly, he told me that he was leaving. I begged, of course. I demanded that he love me. I demanded that he get angry with me. I demanded that he pick up the phone when he left for a four-hour walk.

I told him that I loved him, and I couldn't live without him.

That's when he told me the words that no one wants to hear.

'But, Ally, I don't love you.'

This was the last time I ever begged a man to love me.

THIS TIME, I DIDN'T RUN

As I have discovered while writing this book, when the going gets tough, Ally gets going. I am not a careless runner, but I am someone who will instantly and dramatically exit stage left. Before our relationship *actually* ended, I realised that we were both engineering the end.

I never nudged Tom to read the 'Becoming Ally' post. On some level, I hoped he would be curious about MRKH, and be proud or intrigued about the person I *could* become. Our ten-year relationship had been built on lies and secrecy. Lies that eroded any potential we could have had as a couple. However, it was too late to fix this massive wedge between us. It was time to live a life apart; to find true love and safety.

This time, however, I chose not to run, even though every muscle in my body told me to go – back to England, back to family, anywhere. For so long, I had been blaming anything but myself for my behaviour and where I ended up.

How dare I be born without a vagina?

How dare I be robbed of the experience of growing a child?

How dare the only option for me to have a sexual relationship be to push objects into my 'pouch of a pussy'.

To this point, my unhappiness was not my fault, it was Mother Nature's or science – anyone else's fault but mine. Goddammit, I was owed BIG TIME.

But, blame became relentless.

I could no longer be a passenger in life, waiting for a refund that was never owed to me in the first place. I would enter a relationship with an invisible disclaimer: I am sorry for being defective, thank you for taking me on and I will do my utmost to remain quiet and accept any harm or punishment that you deem fit for me.

This time was different.

So, I didn't beg Tom to take me back.

I didn't pack a bag.

I stayed in the home that was once ours and was now mine.

I was 10,000 miles away from home, single for the first time in 16 years and paying rent for a Bondi apartment I couldn't afford. I was, however, surprisingly hopeful, which was an entirely new feeling. I kept coming back to one question, over and over again: are you prepared, Ally, to be the hero of your story?

PART THREE
Turning the tables on trauma

CHAPTER 9

Enough was enough

If we are lucky enough, we will all get a chance to create a different life, away from the one that has harmed us the most. This usually occurs, however, because we have encountered rock bottom.

We will all have our versions of what rock bottom looks and feels like. For some, it's seeing the bathroom floor every night as you curl up in tears. For others, it will be sitting quietly in a relationship with a person you once loved who is now a stranger.

Sometimes, even rock bottom has a basement.

Sadly, not everyone recovers from a rock-bottom scenario – perhaps a life of addiction and self-harm has overruled a possibility to escape.

Many people sit in their pain because they don't know a way out. Their depression is like sitting in a thick fog day after day. For many, it's being at the hands of violence, with an empty bank account and no salvation to run to. Instead, we tell ourselves a story to attempt to handle depression a little easier: 'Ah well, it could be worse.'

Truly, could it?

Could anything be worse than living a life that causes daily pain? I don't think so. In fact, I know so. It's weird to write, but rock bottom is a destination that can be a blessing – a place we should seek out if we truly want to recover.

If you have lived in the grip of grief, self-hatred, eating disorders, self-medication and/or torrid encounters, rock bottom can take years to find.

For me, while the existence of my rock bottom was a series of toxic relationships, messy acts and living in a body that I couldn't connect to, I came to understand that it was my time to live. I needed to form a relationship with my MRKH diagnosis. I needed to understand the power I had given it, because I identified so strongly with my diagnosis, as opposed to being alongside it.

I no longer wanted to delete Facebook posts. I no longer wanted to negotiate with an unhappy relationship; a sexless, loveless and ungrateful relationship that I know hurt Tom too.

Someone, somewhere, 'up there' – whatever form of heaven I believed in at the time – was handwriting a note. This note was perhaps from the universe, from God, from something greater than me. It was time for me to discover who Ally was all along.

LET'S DISCOVER OUR 'WOO-WOO' WOMANHOOD!

With red eyes and sunken shoulders, I strolled up the hill to my home yoga studio, to flow the grief away. Wearing a pair of cheap, see-through yoga pants (you know, the kind where people can see your knickers, but you haven't twigged that they can yet), I strolled into the studio heavy and sad.

Yoga teachers are massively underappreciated. Weirdly, and beautifully, they become pre- and post-class therapists, to those needing to offload a difficult day.

'Ally, how are you?' said Lennie behind the desk.

'I'm a bit rough. I have just broken up with my boyfriend. And I don't know how I am going to cope.'

Her comforting eyes looked back at me as she too explained that she had just ended a relationship. I felt instant relief. Someone else was getting this sick, shaky and terrifying feeling of being alone. I asked her how long her relationship had been.

'Probably five, maybe six months. You?' she asked.

'Me? Erm, ten years!'

A colleague at work once said to me, 'Ally, here is a little piece of advice. By no means is this a warning but, in fact, a magical gift if you need it to be. Once you discover yoga, be prepared for your life to change.' That was just a short time before Tom and I chose to end our ten-year relationship.

Like most people in the 'Bondi Bubble' – the spiritual mecca that grips onto life's little misfits and wanderers like me – I had discovered Bikram yoga. Situated in Bondi Junction was a studio that pumped 40-degree heat and humidity into a 60-person space. It smelt a little odd, like a combination of sweaty feet and fearlessness. My friend and I were two newbies, eager to pop our 'yoga-cherry'. As we rolled out our flannel-size towels, severely overdressed in T-shirts and running pants, we smiled at each other, awaiting the blissful yoga buzz.

Here's what I didn't know. Bikram yoga isn't exactly what I had pictured. Where were the hippies in floaty tops, embracing their third-eye chakra and being all trippy 'n' shit? Why couldn't I hear the pan pipes on the sound system or smell the incense that would remind me of Bali? Why was everyone who practised before us bright red, dripping in sweat, looking like they lived on a bus?

Fuck. This wasn't the yoga I had in mind.

Even though my friend was clearly hating being ordered through the 26-posture sequence, I was loving it. Immediately I was hooked. This was my version of boot camp for delinquents. I was in a space where my staying power was being challenged. My unloved body was contorting into positions of strength and flexibility that I had no idea I could do.

Sure, my boobs were squashed, flopped and squeezed between my chin and the floor, but I was in heaven. For the first time, I was discovering what it was to finally champion myself. But no sooner was I a Bikram addict than I had developed ravaging eczema overnight, caused by the intense heat in the yoga studio. In the end, my towel was covered in blood from when I would claw at my legs mid-practice. I was in pain and riddled. My Bikram days were over, but my yoga life had just begun. On a search for a new yoga home, I found a cute little studio called YogaBliss tucked away underneath banana leaves and wind chimes. At first, I only signed up for one class, not sure if I'd like it or belong there.

This studio would become my home-from-home for the next five years. This sanctuary would witness my breakdowns, break-ups and breakthroughs. One day it would become my workplace – a nook that was the birthplace for everything I have proudly created, from friendships to self-discoveries; it's the place that I owe my life to in many ways.

ONE EMAIL CAN CHANGE YOUR LIFE

Before Tom and I broke up, I sent an email to a renowned women's hospital in Sydney, which I thought could help me. Understanding that both a London and Boston hospital had successfully created support networks for those with MRKH, I knew I had to get up close and personal with my diagnosis. I knew it wouldn't be easy, but I knew it was time.

After sending a small, brief message to the 'submit option' of their website, not knowing where my email would land, I got an instant reply. The CEO of the women's hospital explained to me that my email had been forwarded to an obstetrician and gynaecology consultant.

Then the big news came.

As I opened my email, my life was to change forever.

Ally, thank you so much for your kind email. It's so incredible that you have reached out to seek support for your MRKH diagnosis. We are so eager to ensure that our patients receive the best treatment and care possible. However, we have not yet established an MRKH support group at the hospital, but we certainly would like to. We would love for you to come for a meeting, and discuss with us your needs as a patient with MRKH, and your thoughts on helping establish an MRKH support group for women in Australia.

Overnight, I was going from a victim to a survivor, and I was about to discover the true power of my pain, if I used a little magic wisely. I thought to myself, 'My gosh, if I am to be part of the change, I need to feel the change in me, too.' For the first time, I experienced a feeling I had never had before.

I felt proud of myself.

I felt hope.

I felt that I had woken up from an emotional coma.

I felt like, for the first time, I was meeting Ally.

The thing about life is that, while we all need to feel a sense of control – to map out our lives from marriage, to children, careers, holidays, bank savings and mealtimes – we are so incredibly powerless. Too much rigidity can cause disappointment. Too much control can rob us of spontaneity. Too much expectation can be the thief of happiness.

WHEN I DISCOVERED AMY, I DISCOVERED A NEW LIFE

You are going to hear about Amy a lot in the second half of this book. In fact, you are going to hear that most of the influential women in my life are, in fact, a bunch of beautiful Amys.

I want to let you in on a little something.

While Amy is the editor of this book, Amy is also my best friend. Actually, she is a 'little twin flame' flickering in the chapters of my life. You could say the day our arms crossed, so did our destined paths. I met Amy at YogaBliss during an afterwork yoga class. There was something special about that studio, in case you hadn't guessed it. It was intimate, 'perfectly imperfect', and seemed to welcome women who appreciated quiet creativity and impromptu chats.

I met Amy by chance when we physically collided. One day, our arms got tangled when reaching for something – our shoes perhaps. Amy apologised for sweeping her sweaty and 'lived-in' trainers under my nose! Upon hearing her English accent, I gravitated towards it with intrigue – who is this beautiful blonde mess?

It was a few weeks before we bumped into each other again. As we stood around in the reception area, I overheard her talking to another student. She mentioned that she was a journalist – an editor at a fashion magazine. When I heard this, I immediately decided I just had to speak to her. It seemed meant to be.

I had to ask for her help in bringing awareness to the forefront of Australian media with my passion project (my life, in fact) of MRKH advocacy. And that I did. Emails were exchanged, countless chai dates in corner cafés were had, and soon, really soon, she became, gosh, my closest friend.

It was only a matter of time before our weekly catch-up became daily purges about relationships, love, life and all the truly crappy bits that can come with being a woman in their early thirties, in the middle of this huge and magnetic metropolis.

The thing about Amy is that she is a powerful storyteller. She is unafraid to venture into the topics that most tiptoe around. Amy understands trauma in a way that is safe and unassuming. With a crazy ability to understand the way we tick as humans, Amy's words can heal the hardest and hurt of hearts.

As an author and woman with her own adverse backstory, Amy was ahead of her time as a writer, long before I met her. She believed in the power of truth-telling and handling trauma with so much care that we can heal safely. We can own the parts of us that most will filter out. We can give ourselves permission to be bravely un-brave, despite pop culture telling us that being resilient is every woman's most crucial resource.

You probably can tell I am crazy about our friendship. Yes, Amy, I am crazy about you!

When I met Amy, I didn't realise at the time that she was six years into being widowed. Just three weeks after she married the man of her dreams, he passed away from terminal and recurrent cancer. As a gifted and determined survivor, Amy wrote her first book aged just 23, about a widow who grieved in a different way.

She didn't want to dress head to toe in black or commit to the grieving rules expected of her. So, she did healing in a different way. Amy's debut memoir, *Wife, Interrupted*, tells the story of how she overcame her bereavement by having uncomplicated sex with men around London. She stood behind her truth then, and I suspect she has never stopped since. Because if we can't speak our truth, we are doing our soul an absolute disservice.

I read Amy's book in two days. I needed to understand who Amy was, and what she had been through, if I was going to be a friend worth keeping. And I am not too shy to say that there may have been a little idolisation at first. And for good reason too. (I'm OK with that, if you are, Amy?)

Seriously, I need to gush a little.

When I broke up with Tom, she didn't offer me a typical list of 'how to get over the guy' anecdotes: 'plenty more fish in the sea, Ally', 'jump on a dating app, Ally', 'better off without him, Ally'.

Nup. Amy understood that while the relationship was so wrong for me, I was allowed to miss a person who had been in my life for a decade. There was no judgement, no advice, or activities on how to live my #bestlife.

There was, however, something sitting on my doorstep as I returned home one day.

Wrapped in flashy paper, with a tag that read 'Ally, everyone deserves pleasure. Enjoy.'

Yep, Amy had bought me a vibrator, despite knowing my diagnosis and my history.

MEETING MY OTHER BABY

When Amy and I met, she was in a huge life transition too. She had just met a guy she'd fallen head over heels in love with, after only a few weeks of meeting him. It was the kind of fast romance that people easily criticise (do they really know what they're doing?). Amy, however, doesn't take on other people's opinions. Within a year of Amy and I meeting, they were engaged – and she asked me to be her bridesmaid.

When Amy asked me to be by her side during her wedding, I cried happy, happy tears. We all deserve love, but by geez, this lady really deserves long-lasting love that will bring her the magic milestones we grow up hoping for.

The morning of Amy's wedding, post-breakfast and pre-make-up, the wedding party gathered for a surprise announcement. I knew what it was before we even pulled up to the house. They were pregnant.

As an infertile woman, I knew this day would come. The day our best friends commence a journey we long for, and the conflict soon dawns on us that while we want to be privy to every twinge, bump and vaginal discovery (cue, mucus plug) that comes with pregnancy, we also know that in contrast, we are staring our nemesis in the eye.

Fertile or not, most – not every, but most – people will assume that one day they will become parents, or at least factor family planning into life's big decisions. When I was a child, I would play with Barbie dolls, a styling-head doll and a doll that even soiled itself. From a child to the time I was diagnosed with MRKH, I thought becoming a mother was a given. I'd meet a man, fall in love with him and start a family. Rarely are we taught anything else as children by school science classes and society.

Even upon learning that I wouldn't ever be able to carry a child biologically, I always hoped I would one day have a daughter. The imagery of this blonde-haired, blue-eyed and dainty little girl would drift in and out of my imagination. She was so real.

When I took my corporate job in Sydney, I was on seriously good money, as was Tom. I would always take charge of the savings account. I took great satisfaction in seeing my bank balance soar. So did Tom, but I had a different agenda. The money in our joint savings account was not just for fancy holidays and Bondi Beach rent, it was for my secret plan, my baby.

I have never really felt myself as clucky. I would have the odd burst of broodiness, but I didn't gravitate towards children at birthday parties or park picnics. Part of me feared that other parents would see the invisible A-board hanging over my shoulders: 'I'm the girl who can't have children. Protect your precious cargo.' However, that was my issue, not theirs.

So, deep, deep down, I was planning the arrival of my baby. Deep, deep down I was imagining the delivery room as I heard her cry for the first time. Deep, deep down I was envisaging her holding her hand out to me, with love. Deep, deep down I wanted my parents to love my child.

Deep, deep down, quietly and hopefully, I was plotting to make myself a mother.

Infertility: it's not fair or unfair. It's not to be pitied or disregarded, and it is the invisible grief that most will never talk about. The inner dialogue for infertility is that of subtle sadness, disguised aggression and palpable fear. Whether you ever desired to be a parent or not is quite irrelevant – but when you are questioning the evolutionary pothole in the road that threatens empty Christmases or not feeling 'that kick' for the first time, there is only one thing to do – and that's talk about it.

To do this without a 'how-to guide', or indeed obvious envy, challenges everything we have learnt as young, intelligent and apparently prepared women.

In the coming months, I would learn the honest and unedited truths that come with pregnancy – morning sickness, mood changes and leaking boobs. A few days before she gave birth, Amy sent me a photograph of her 'mucus plug' (you don't want to Google it!). Long story short, I never felt excluded.

In fact, I was learning. It was truly fascinating, but then, as the due date was approaching, I started to feel weird, a little nervous. I felt myself feeling – can I say it? – a little sad.

Can I dare, dare say it – a little jealous?

I was so scared I was going to lose her. I was so scared that Mother Nature's natural divide would keep Amy from being part of my life and that I wouldn't be able to relate to her anymore – worst still, that her giving birth would validate that I am not a full and worthy woman. Would I lose my best friend?

You only have to scroll through a Facebook feed to see a thread of baby scan pictures and engagement photos. Despite my love and happiness for Amy and her family, I felt not only physically lacking, but emotionally terrified.

I believe there are two things I am not meant to do – drive a car and hold a baby. It's a weird conclusion I have drawn up for myself –

but part of me feels that perhaps if I was born without a womb, I was born without the instinct to hold something so precious safely.

Instead of shying away from the problem, Amy tackled it head-on. One morning, she sent me a YouTube clip on 'How to Hold a Baby'. That was our friendship – honest and upfront. I explained to her that, despite my happiness for her, I was sad for me and worried that my growing disconnect would damage what we have – she was my family here. She was my Amy.

I made her promise that when the baby was coming, she would send me the news in cryptic code (as everything we have done has always been a little quirky and left of centre). My cryptic code would come in the form of an Eighties-themed something or other.

On Friday, 30th September, at 6 a.m., my phone went 'ping!!!'

On my screen appeared a montage of Madonna, Ghostbusters and Michael Jackson.

Her baby – 'our baby' – was on her way.

YOUR CAPACITY TO LOVE

A pillow was laid on my lap and Amy carefully placed her baby in my arms, and I just felt such peace. I felt the well of tears draw up from the back of my throat. I felt every chai tea we had ever ordered manifest into this small, tiny and perfect human being. I felt the love of two people who never felt entitled to it, creating it so naturally. I felt my best friend look down on me, with such delicacy and respect.

And never once did I feel infertile. Never once did I feel envy.

I don't want to be that woman who feels cheated – I don't want to constantly feel like a spectator or an observer of life, unable to have it all.

Pain and loss are all around us, either in the neighbour's apartment or with the girl sitting next to us on a train – we are all feeling like something is a little missing.

Fertility is at the core of who we are, and some would even go as far as to say it's why we are here. And as for the infertile, while our peers mould into neat families, there is always someone feeling a little bit lonely, like us.

Find them and be their friend.

True healing does not just come in time.

True healing is not something you learn just on a yoga mat or in a therapist's chair.

I was healing as I kissed this newborn's nose-tip, because I knew that love is only one 'blonde mess' away.

SHE NEARLY DIED, TO SHOW ME HOW TO SURVIVE

When you choose to live in Australia instead of the UK, you choose to live far away from family. It's a trade-off for a life in the iconic Bondi Beach. However, sometimes the circumstances were different. With vast time zones and poor reception in my apartment, my weekly phone calls home were lean and more about sharing facts than feelings.

For expats, their biggest fear is 'the midnight phone call' – the phone call from their motherland with terrible news. If you're lucky, you'll go a decade living here without receiving one. I wasn't so lucky.

Just months after I split up from Tom, the phone call came. At 4 a.m., I was shocked out of my sleep by the ringing. As soon as I saw my brother's name light up my screen, I knew that I was about to experience the most gut-wrenching phone call of my life.

In tears, he slowly said, 'It's Mum. She is in hospital.' After a pause, which felt like a lifetime, he continued, 'She's had a stroke.'

I couldn't quite breathe.

I had only spoken to her six hours before. I knew she was under a little stress, but she's Mum, she's strong, and young, and healthy.

I knew that strokes can be so unbiased in who they target. But this couldn't be happening. Not to her.

It was possibly the longest flight of my life. I sat for 23 hours, not knowing if the person I loved the most was dying without me. My dad embraced me at Heathrow, as he always does. He reassured me that she was going to be OK. Even today, when he sees pain in my eyes, he will do whatever it takes to make sure that he carries the weight, if it means I don't have to.

When I walked into the hospital room to see my mum, I expected the worst. Would I even recognise her? Her mouth was slightly dropped to the right, but aside from that, she was Mum. We hugged for what felt like hours. I was relieved, but at the same time, I had experienced unimaginable fear.

The fear of knowing that I will never escape the reality of losing someone I love. The fear of knowing my life was just beginning, on the opposite side of the world. The fear of realising that in a moment, life can be so rapidly interrupted.

Ten days later, my mum was sitting at home, a different woman. Brain injuries can affect not only the mobility of a body, but also a person's emotional state. For days and weeks, she learnt how to read again, and read aloud. A trick I picked up in yoga, to 'follow your Drishti', meaning 'to focus and gaze' in Sanskrit, helped her walk in a straight and steady line.

This, the most significant turnaround moment in my entire life, was being delivered yet again by my soulmate, my beautiful Mama – the person who has never stopped teaching me what it truly is to survive.

When I left Australia in a panic after the phone call, I had no idea how long I'd be gone. My job had given me 'compassionate leave', so I wasn't in a rush to return. While Mum recovered from her trauma, I felt like it was an absolute injustice to her recovery if I wasn't prepared to do the same. I needed to shed my victim status and start taking true responsibility for my happiness – whatever that was to look like.

After one month in England, with both of us nursing our wounds, I knew it was time to go back to Australia. As I boarded the plane to Sydney, I felt a shift. I was ready to commit to my life there and this new version of myself.

Sometimes, the only way we know it's time to heal is because there is nothing left to break.

CHAPTER 10

My pain becomes my superpower

As the taxi pulled into the front entrance at the Sydney hospital, I had one phone call to make, back to my UK home, to my mum. In just a matter of moments, I would step into a conference room to co-host Australia's first MRKH Support Group event. They say that to begin to overcome grief, an important step is to find meaning in what you've been through.

'Mum, I can't believe today has come. I cannot believe that I have run for so long away from my body, away from my voice, for my entire adult life. And now I am here.'

Here I was – a womb-less person who had to make her own vagina. And I am not going to claim that any of it was OK. Not the abuse, the self-harm, the drunken months on strangers' floors. But here I was: a survivor, a speaker, a change-maker.

As I walked through the hospital doors, I thought to myself, 'Today, I get to tell my story. A story that, until now, had no meaning. Was I actually meant to have MRKH all along?'

The last few months of preparation for this meeting had pushed me to my limits, especially as I was still working on it around my full-time job. It's amazing what you can achieve when you're single, childless and driven by trauma.

I went from patient to advocate. I went from destruction to demonstrator. I went from harmed to home, as I found my place back on this earth again. Joined by a team of Australian experts, we drafted, tweaked and created a day that was solely designed to embrace and hold a safe space for those who, like me, were diagnosed with MRKH.

After months of preparation, hospital meetings and taking the calls of tentative attendees, we had crafted a campaign that would change the national footprint in women's health.

'Today, I will share my story for the first time as a public speaker.'

My hands shook as I stood at the microphone in front of a group of women – women who'd been directed here by their doctors, their therapists, their specialists and their peers. Some arrived with their mothers, some arrived alone. Some spoke of their trauma, while others cried at the back of the room. For hours, their pain was our purpose, to make meaning of, and to uncover what it means to be 'different'.

I didn't try to hide my nerves, instead I gave them a reason to trust me.

'I am just like you. I am still where you are. We can all get through this diagnosis together.'

MY VAGINA WENT PUBLIC

I need to preface this chapter by saying I don't believe that the word vagina needs to be flung around just for the sake of it. There is always a time, place and context for talking about 'what happens down there'. For me, I knew that if I was going to be an advocate of my word, then I couldn't tell half-truths. I couldn't just talk about what society finds acceptable and comfortable.

Today, infertility is talked about openly (as it should be). We see pictures on billboards and media advertising about top-notch IVF clinics and how 'the family dream' can be achieved. Typically, there is a man and woman, clutching their newborn, thanks to the pioneering IVF clinics and science that have made the impossible possible.

But, what about sexual dysfunction?

Now, in my mid-thirties, that side of sexuality and procreation was still hidden in shadows.

And what about vaginas?

When do they get a look-in (societally, not literally – for me, that has been seen in plentiful measures!)?

Infertility and sexual function are two very different topics. If women, however, cannot express their fear, their pain and the 'unspeakable', how are they ever going to heal their traumas? If we don't explain the process of vaginal dilation, sexual dysfunction, decades of silencing by the awkwardness of others, we are no longer just carrying our pain but society's too.

This is why I knew that my story and the method behind my advocacy was to challenge the norms, get creative with my storytelling techniques and hold my nerve when it came to public and personal disclosures.

With the success of the hospital event, I knew that this life was in fact designed for me. I was born into this body to tell this story. I was meant to have MRKH. My story was hard enough to help me understand MRKH and healed enough to help me challenge it.

One thing I knew, however, was I didn't want to do it alone. I had spent so much of my life feeling alone – not fitting in or belonging. I wanted a partner, a friend and community builder by my side. There was one woman who stood out to me at the MRKH Support Group event.

Her name was Lucy.

After being connected to Lucy before the big day, we spoke of her journey to parenthood. She and her husband had travelled to India to see the birth of their daughter with a gestational surrogate. We spoke openly about the thousands of dollars they spent, the heartache they experienced and the emotional toll of becoming a mother without a uterus.

Instantly, I knew Lucy was the person I wanted by my side to launch Australia's first MRKH foundation. With wildly blonde hair, a heart that was built of pure love and an edginess I adored, she was something special.

That day, the Sisters for Love MRKH Foundation, which would later be rebranded, was launched. Before landing on this one, I am embarrassed to say that names didn't come easy to me. I teetered between 'The Mango Tree' (I have absolutely no idea what mangoes have to do with vaginas) and 'The Healing Hub' (kinda catchy, but equally as irrelevant to girl talk).

What I did know was that a unique sisterhood existed in the MRKH community, and what all of us want is to feel love; from others and, ultimately, ourselves.

IF IT FEELS EASY, IT'S RIGHT

For years, I felt like a serial failure; I failed at relationships, education, jobs, positive sexual intimacy and life generally. I would graze from relationship to relationship and follow the lead of others. I would sit on the sidelines, waiting and hoping for the happiness to start.

Self-doubt was a daily feeling and I accepted that success would come in my 'next life'.

However, building the Sisters for Love MRKH Foundation fell into place. By no means was it easy. I would spend every spare hour building websites, creating content, sending emails to hospitals across

Australia, and mentoring those who found our Facebook page. Every night, I would schedule calls with people diagnosed with MRKH.

Some were teenagers, and some were in their late sixties. I would cram myself into the corner of my apartment (because Bondi has zero reception) and chat to people for hours about their diagnosis day. I would spend hours commenting on Facebook forums and soon became one of the most active in the MRKH world.

Influenced and inspired by an American support group called the Beautiful You MRKH Foundation, I reached out to its founders, Amy and Christina. I started to know who's who in the advocacy zoo. I started to feel like I could make an impact in my corner of the world.

After years of isolation, I was now spending every waking minute building and creating campaigns to get the word out there. At first, I believed the way to put us on the Australian map was to create a charity. But I soon realised that was not a goal I should be chasing. Funds at this point were not necessary. What became instantly apparent was that no one knew what 'MRKH' stood for, medical professionals included.

Our mission was to talk about, write, share, promote and put ourselves on the media circuit to explain what these four lone letters mean. Interestingly, some took the bait immediately. In the early days, I would go in gently: 'I can't possibly put the word "vagina" into a subject heading, can I?'

Apparently, that's what was going to get us noticed. It was a respectful juggle between telling the truth, but not making the diagnosis into a circus act. We know the power of a hook, a clickbait headline, but ... I was learning that me and my vagina needed to go public.

Buckle-up, inhale, exhale and tell the truth.

There was only one way we were going to find freedom from our 'flight' response and that was to be intelligently disruptive.

It wasn't long before we hosted our second and then third MRKH Support Group at the Sydney hospital. Year on year, it just kept getting bigger and better. Clinical specialists were flying in to make presentations, surrogacy experts were sharing the processes to intended parents, and scientific researchers wanted to partner with us to discover the gene mutation behind MRKH.

I had only ever attended one support group event and that was at my treatment hospital in London. I remember listening to one clinical psychologist speak – how gentle her voice was and how well she understood my anger and shame. I was so angry, in fact, that I stormed out, with my mum wondering what had triggered me to leave halfway through the day. My teenage voice was full of pain:

'I don't want to fucking be here. It's full of people talking about their feelings. It's full of people smiling with hopeful bullshit. That's not real life. Real life is pain, cuts and eating disorders. Real life is tubes, lubes and a broken body. I'm done.'

Nearly twenty years later, as I planned another support group, I remembered this memory. After a tip-off from a doctor, I discovered that, amazingly, this psychologist now lived near Sydney. It seemed meant to be! With some digging, I found her contact details. On a wing and a prayer, I sent her what was less like an email, and more like a long-lost letter of gratitude and apology.

Just months later, we were reunited at our next MRKH conference. We understood professional boundaries, so we didn't hug it out, but our eyes did the talking. She remembered me and how I wasn't ready for help. She remembered me abruptly leaving the room all those years ago.

Yet, here we were, 10,000 miles and 17 years away from our first introduction, making waves on Australian soil.

In time, advocacy will find you, before you find it. There is a calling that feels magical and powerful. It's a calling that becomes a responsibility and, in some ways, becomes your greatest purpose. It's a contract you make with the universe, and an apology to your past. It feels like forgiveness and a second chance. It also becomes an administration marathon.

WHAT IF MY DATE GOOGLES ME?

Finding myself single for the first time in nearly 17-something years was weird. Weird and wonderful. I knew I was in safe hands, as I explained to Amy how petrified I was to put my toe in the Bondi dating pool ... which, by the way, felt like a shark fest (no pun intended!).

Cue, dating apps. Just, eugh! I never liked them, but that didn't stop me scrolling on my daily commute to my bill-paying job; that's the term advocates use when distinguishing between our financial income and soul-purpose role (advocacy). I would put up cute profiles, and call myself the 'red-wine sipping, ocean-frolicking, sandy-footed yogi'. It sounded good at the time!

My first match was with a doctor, and I was like, 'This is easy!!' Here comes the (unhelpful) storytelling us gals can do when our imagination runs away with itself. I instantly thought, 'Well, this is it. I'm going to marry a doctor; we will change women's health across the nation and it won't be long before I am in a committed relationship again.'

I sent him a message full of excitement and then waited for his response. Yep, nup. Nothing, nada!

I was beginning to realise this dating thing wouldn't be easy, even with thousands of potential matches in my smartphone. Plus, there was the disclosure element. I wasn't a girl with a hidden diagnosis anymore. I was an out-there advocate for my diagnosis.

Here I was talking to rooms of patients and doctors, conducting media interviews, and sharing the latest news across social media platforms. But looking into the eyes of a single person, and a stranger, transports me and my courage back to the early days.

What on earth was I going to say if someone asked me about children, family planning or what I do in my spare time?

Fuck, the disclosure part is here AGAIN!

My biggest fear was being googled, like one particular date did after we met.

I could tell instantly that something was wrong when we sat down for a romantic night for two. He was cold, distant and avoiding eye contact. So, I mustered the courage and asked him if anything was wrong.

'Ally, it's all a bit weird,' he said. 'How do I know that you won't go off the rails again? How do I know if we could ever have a family?' By date number five, this short-lived romance was over. While he never came out and actually said the words, 'I don't want to be with you because of your diagnosis and rocky past,' I knew that I wasn't the person for him.

I knew that he wanted a bona fide family with children in his future, and I could not guarantee any of that. To say I was crushed is a massive understatement.

I understand that we all get intrigued by a person we are potentially going to date. I didn't, however, want someone to read an article on the internet and decide who I am or what it means to be in a relationship with me.

What will they think of me?

Will they see me as a freak?

When is it too soon to share that I'm infertile?

I didn't want to lead anyone up the garden path, but discussing babies, infertility and IVF options over a sunset margarita seemed a little premature. And, what happens if I explain the 'why' behind my lack of oven for any impending bun? I would have to say M-R-K-H, give my 'elevator pitch' about my condition and explain 'the vagina thing is all good here, and in complete working order'.

There is sexy talk and there is sex talk – and the two are *very* different.

I do believe, when you're hiding something from a partner – even just a dinner date – they tend to sense it. So, rarely would I get past date number five. Maybe I made it that way, maybe it just wasn't meant to be.

At the same time, I was dating myself. That sounds a bit naff, but it's true. I didn't know what pleasure or true reciprocal desire felt like. I didn't know what I wanted from a relationship or what I had to give. For many who have experienced trauma in any form, understanding love is a process that deserves kindness and reflection.

We don't always know the damage our pasts have done, until we sample our present. We don't know the worth that has been chipped away, until we need to use it. The memories of abuse, harm and self-disgust need to be forgiven, before we can honour new ones into our lives.

For the first time in my life, I was sampling self-love. Like any relationship, it was scary, unknown and consuming.

Self-love is a term we scroll over often, but it can mean something different for everyone. After being in a relationship for pretty much my entire adult life, self-love was a foreign concept. Some days gave me simple, solo joys like swimming in the ocean all day without a curfew or sitting in the sunshine writing alone. Other days, I would revel in being able to eat what I wanted and go make my plans without seeking permission.

Then, self-love was all about exploring my body. I would see the way my body was changing after racking up eight classes of yoga a week. Not to mention, perfectly orgasming daily with me, myself and I. Booking last-minute flights for long weekends in Byron Bay, or simply sitting in meditation with the Sydney sun pitching down on my balcony. These were effortless moments of liberation.

For the first time, I was answerable to no one. There was no judgement, rules or remorse for living selflessly.

My life was for my advocacy work and myself. And that was a pretty unbeatable date night.

CHAPTER 11

Do relationships ever really end?

There is always a murky shade of grey between the break-up and going 'no contact' with an ex. After all, I was with Tom for ten years of my life and some heart habits are tricky to break. While I didn't beg Tom to stay, I wasn't completely ready to let him vanish out of my life either. I knew the relationship was a pile of rubble and neither of us wanted it. We both wanted to invent new lives apart; however, I was still having issues when it came to boundaries.

It had been eight months since we broke up and I still relied on my ex a lot. Tom always completed our yearly tax returns, so when tax season hit, I asked him for help. Holidays that we'd planned together before we broke up remained in our diaries and neither of us cancelled them. Our bank accounts were linked and so were our pasts.

At one point, Tom wanted me to meet his new girlfriend, so our friendship didn't have to end. After an emergency phone call to Amy, we both agreed that a trio meet-up was probably not the best idea. I didn't want Tom to vanish, but I didn't want him to stay either. If I am being brutally honest with myself, I didn't want to know how easily he had fallen in love when I was nowhere close to it. Part of me didn't want to see how happy he was, because I would have been reminded of how sad I made him. If only the heart didn't feel guilt.

The tug-of-war in any break-up stems from holding on to the last thread of regret. Regret for the pain that was felt in the relationship, for it not working, and for holding on, when we should have let go sooner. Even now, eleven years later, Tom and I swap 'happy birthday' messages. I still go to him for financial advice, despite knowing I could easily find the information on my own. There is a bond that will always remain between us. And with any ex, I guess, because memories you can't undo. I make it a goal of mine (unless the toxicity is too untreatable) to never have bad blood with an ex, despite the shit-show that some relationships were. Not even with James, who physically abused me. While we don't have any contact, I know that he knew it was time to end our toxic relationship. I saw a desire in him to heal, and I cannot fault that, as strange as it may seem to other people.

I knew that, before making a future that was right for me, I needed to discover why the past wasn't right.

HOW TO REPURPOSE OUR PAIN

In the year after breaking up with Tom, I became a trauma observer – like a zoologist studying a species. I was fascinated by what made people hurt, helped people recover and enabled some people to rise from despair, while others drowned in it.

I gravitated towards 'tell-all books' written by women who had overcome trauma and adversity. My bed stand had a stack of memoirs authored by women who, at a young age, found themselves in the depths of despair, because doesn't that make us all feel better? I was also drawn to those kinds of conversations, whether with friends or strangers.

A friend once said to me, 'Ally, you don't befriend people unless they've had a dark past.' I immediately took offence at that comment, fearing that I was a sucker for a dramatic ending. In fact, I have never stopped unpicking that comment. The last thing I want to be is someone who craves pain and drama. No one wants to be *that* girl.

As I continued to wade through this thing called life, I didn't seek out people who had a dark past – I sought out people who found a way to survive. I found comfort, relatability and safety in people who refused to sit in silence with my truth. I wanted to sit in theirs. I didn't just want to, I *needed* to be as close to the truth as possible, because I knew what happened when I didn't.

I had been a self-harmer and a toxic relationship migrator. I had disappeared into drunken crowds and smacked a smile on a broken heart. But most of all, I had denied myself a chance at living life without shame.

Today, I am an avid truth teller – it's even become my profession. I want us, women, and men, to be gentle with hearts and fearless with our pain. I want every human who has sat in a body that has no drop-down menu to select from, or category on a medical form, to discover the soul that sits behind the skin.

First, we must hunt out our wounds and go back to the beginning to where it all started. My advice, before you throw on your backpack towards your soul adventure, is to find a friend who can hold you at each discovery point; a home that feels like a home, with an abundance of self-compassion, because you, lovely, are so worth it.

THE BULLSHIT ABOUT BOUNDARIES

If you could see my face at this exact moment, you would see a gentle smile. Why? Because I love chatting about all things boundaries, despite once not knowing what they truly meant.

I could write a whole book about boundaries, despite there being hundreds published already. I encourage you to have at least one boundary-themed book in your collection. It's only taken me, hmmm, 40 years or so, to relish and relate to the idea of boundaries, because I finally get them.

Boundaries: I have loathed them and now I love them.

How weird and brilliant is that?

Lovely boundaries are everyone's best friend (if, hopefully, you accept their 'friend request').

There is nowhere in the human psyche where boundaries don't deserve a shout-out. They belong in friendships, romantic trysts, workplaces, sex, divorce, family holidays, money loans and even books.

Yes, this book has been one big boundary negotiation. Should I write that? Should I share that secret? Should I go into *that* much detail? Am I sharing enough? Am I protecting the people I love? How much of the truth should I share?

Boundaries have this bold yet delicate way of needing to be part of every decision we make. Boundaries protect us and the people we love, acting as an emotional flyscreen between us and the boundary.

When we have boundaries in place, we can 'see pain, but not feel pain'. We can love someone hugely, but we can love ourselves more. We can make a lifelong marriage work if an early boundary chat takes place.

For me, boundaries for a long time were non-existent.

Throughout many of my relationships, speaking up was speaking out. I felt that if I asked for my needs to be met, I was appearing needy. If I wanted more sex, I was a slut. If I wanted less sex, I was a prude. If I wanted more money, I was greedy. If I wanted a fulfilling job, I was relentless. If I wanted structure, I was bored.

Boundaries are, in fact, there to enable happiness and not rob it.

If you are sitting on a hard-and-fast life-changing event, understand the protective shield you have in place. Believe that you owe your happiness to this choice. But whatever you do, never ignore that voice in your gut. If it feels wrong, it likely isn't the best choice for you.

Boundaries, instincts and worth are your biggest cheerleaders in the pro-you camp.

Welcome in boundaries like you would the love of your life, because in many ways, boundaries are going to either make or break a brighter day.

A PAIN CYCLE THAT I HAD TO BREAK

I am going to say what I may have said before – pain is actually a good thing. One night recently, I accidentally snipped the tip of my thumb off preparing dinner. It was one of those 'out-of-body experiences', where I saw my manicured thumbnail clinging to a fairly decent chunk of flesh.

The blood was pouring, my nail was waving in the wind (slight exaggeration! Let's say hanging limply on the offending knife). I was wondering, 'What the fuck am I going to do?' Of course, I didn't think to call the emergency services, I texted a friend. The pain was being nicely disguised by shock and I felt sending a WhatsApp message was a better move than seeking professional help!

Unexpected harm during a self-harming recovery can be extremely scary. I was a pro at pain but it comes down to control. I had no control over this mishap and I was not prepared for the surge of pain that came overnight as I lay in bed, bandaged up, wondering if I was going to be thumbless.

So, instead of hating the pain, I understood that it was there to protect me. It was there to buffer my healing from knocks and bumps. My pain was my protector. This increasing agony was the messenger to tell my body that it's under threat. Being the stoic, 'let's not cause a fuss' type of person I am, it took me a week to finally get it checked out. To my surprise, I was 'over-healing'.

What? Can a body do too much healing?

Doesn't this go against everything I have learnt? Ironically, two days before I had cut my finger, Amy and I were chatting about the negative effects of healing, or as she so perfectly put it, 'over-correcting'.

I am going to save this concept for a later chapter revelation, but the point is, pain is good, and yet often we go to extremes to avoid the pain of our pasts. However, the pendulum can sometimes swing so much one way that we avoid opening up our hearts.

All my life, I had participated in pain, but I ran from it the moment my soul should have started its healing process. The soul scars were healing without the treatment they needed. I don't regret my past one bit. However, ignoring the demons is doing an absolute disservice to our pain.

It's a bit like our first messy and brutal break-up. We meet a person who unlocks the feeling of falling in love. Nothing beats the first-love butterflies towards the person we idolise and fantasise about for nights on end. Until our forever person breaks our heart or we break theirs.

Hearts get broken – that's the reality of life. I remember sobbing to my mum after the break-up of my first true love. She did everything to console me. She let me lie and cry in a heap, and listened for hours on end, as I shared my 'how to win him back' tactics.

As the wise woman she is, she explained that 'now you know this pain, it's unlikely you'll feel it like this again'. That's not to say each heartache will get easier, but my heart was prepped a little better, although it didn't feel like it at the time. The trick is, be open to love as if it's a flyscreen and not an iron door. We all know what happens when our walls go up – we deny ourselves those butterflies.

The problem with my 'pain-plan' was that I became more familiar with the part where it damaged me. I had become so immersed in feelings of sadness that I knew no different. I felt more at peace with destruction than I did with remedies. My pain cycle was simple and mastered; hurt, acknowledge, disguise, deny, punish and repeat.

WHAT YOUR PAIN IS TRYING TO TELL YOU

Twelve months after Tom and I broke up, it was finally time to really separate our lives. I knew it was time, Amy kept kindly suggesting it was time, and he was in love and ready to move on with his life.

After Tom and I finally settled our finances and he collected the last of his belongings in our tree-top Bondi apartment, for the first time in my life, I was single. Like, ridiculously single. Tom had been more than fair with splitting our savings in two, and now I am so happy to say that we are friends who have made our amends.

I didn't realise at the time but, ten years later, we'd remain an echo in each other's lives. I will always smile fondly when I think of him. A decade on, I'm so proud and happy for the man he became – happily married and building a home for him and his wife.

It's so important to remember that we are not our pasts. Nothing riles me more than hearing the phrase, 'a leopard can't change its spots', because we as humans have the ability to do anything we want if committed to the process.

This is why forgiveness is part of any break-up, whether it takes months or years to discover. When Tom told me that our relationship was over, I didn't ask or beg him to stay. I didn't plead with him to change his decision. Despite me drinking a bottle of champagne for breakfast the day after it happened, I actually didn't fight the fear. I knew it was over, and not just the relationship.

I was entering a new chapter of my life. Even on my toughest days, I could see this as true. In this way, Amy continued to guide me and inspire me. I needed to be close to a person who had challenged her past and owned up to the behaviours that others will judge. In fact, one saying I stand by is 'he who is without sin, cast the first stone', meaning, if you haven't fucked up in life, sure, take a pop at my problems. Otherwise, allow me the room to be a human. I am always learning.

Slowly, over the course of a few months, I would sit with Amy drinking chai and explore how I wanted to tell my story. I started to talk about my MRKH diagnosis more and more on social media and how it left me feeling like a broken and ashamed person.

We would go to yoga workshops, where I was slowly being introduced to spiritual enthusiasts and those who were also runners from a different life. I stopped wearing long-sleeve shirts in yoga to hide my scars and swapped to tank tops, which showed all of me – my past, my present and my hopes for the future.

That's the thing about the beautiful Bondi Beach, it seems to attract the black sheep of the family; the emotional misfits who need a softer landing to heal.

That's not to say those who were closest to me were not perfect. In my eyes, every human I rolled my mat alongside was their greatest selves. They cried openly, embraced a hug like they meant it, and were creatives on a mission to change a norm. Like me, they were craving something bigger, gentler, kinder and crazier.

I was home.

As a fledgling MRKH advocate, the Sisters for Love MRKH Foundation was thriving.

Together, Lucy and I created an ambassador programme inviting women to represent a handful of Australian states, plus the UK and America. As lovers of digital storytelling, we created a campaign titled, 'A True Reaction: The Sisters for Love Passion Project', which told the unspoken truths of a crippling medical diagnosis.

One day, I sent seven letters, across Australia and the globe, to the foundation's ambassadors. All I asked for was one act of honesty. These letters contained a set of questions that, for any person with MRKH, would be provocative and challenging. I placed one request: press record on your camera first, open the letter second. This emotional campaign delved deep as we discovered the truth about what lies beneath the surface of MRKH.

We were becoming a community that felt so easy to create, because it was right. We raised and rallied thousands of dollars. Researchers would seek us out, and parents and partners would send us messages in their plea for hope and understanding on how to help the person they love. We were changing the landscape of peer support, and I knew that this was all meant for me.

I was dismantling my pain, to build a presence. I was sharing my truth about this diagnosis to the public, to solidify the importance of owning a story that once broke me.

When I wasn't working from 5 p.m. in my corporate job, I was running home to video-call advocates around the globe and talking to those who had never spoken to anyone with MRKH. With every story I heard, I was able to relate to the loneliness that others felt. For the first time, I wasn't circling the outside of a crowd, I was part of one. With every presentation, interview and support group, I took the pain to fuel me. Like a blood transfusion, the pain was coming in, and the purpose was coming in.

As a community of like-minded people, we were repurposing our pain and creating our superpowers. Not always life-altering powers. For some, including myself, it was the power to share my past with a friend, to disclose to a new partner that I was unable to carry children biologically, and the power of forgiveness. It was the power to crack open the honesty box of how I came to the parts of my story that could have ended me, and this bravery was infectious beyond comprehension.

The MRKH community is a collection of courageous people whose lives were rocked the way mine was. A community that would start to tell their stories, raise money for the foundation, brand a T-shirt with the four letters MRKH to raise awareness, and who would never leave a person behind. With every forum post asking a question, 100 responses were shared. With every cry for help, there were 100 women messaging, 'DM me, I am here to talk.' Every email from a doctor was an opportunity to bridge the gap between professional and patient.

We were putting MRKH on the map and, for the first time in my life, I felt hopeful. I was thanking every past pain for showing me the contrast between unhappy and happy. I was making sense of the abuse and silent treatments. I was getting angry at situations that I once should have been angry at, and not complicit in.

I was finally becoming Ally.

I know your story can be told. Take all that pain, throw it in the air and allow it to land in peace. It was never there to haunt you, but to be a compass to the next road you take.

WHEN YOUR VAGINA MAKES THE HEADLINES!

It's a funny feeling when the thing you've been dreaming of happens. I wanted to get MRKH out there and raise awareness; I wanted to be seen, heard and feel like my story matters. Suddenly, the media was paying attention and it was a pivotal moment.

Soon enough, I was reading headlines such as, 'Born Without a Vagina'. Advocate or not, sometimes reading your name against this bold disclosure is pretty hard. I knew that it was my job to post, share and back any publication that was going to offer MRKH a platform. But, geez, did I have oversharer's remorse on a number of occasions.

As the months went on and our profile rose, I would regularly be asked to interview for podcasts, local and national. Sometimes, I would say yes to any story if it meant we could boost our campaign. Working with the media was an experiment in trust. I worried about what people would think about me, when I didn't have a chance to defend the facts (which, actually, were pretty spot on).

Behind closed doors, I was torn between my role as a speaker and a person coming to terms with public exposure. On certain days, despite my public-speaking rituals such as listening to a gee-up soundtrack, wearing my feel-good black shirt and making an SOS call back home, the words didn't always leave my mouth correctly.

Conversely, overconfidence caused me to share a little too much on some occasions. Once, I listened back to an 'overconfident podcast'. By no means is there anything wrong with overconfidence, but consistency is key. As I drew the curtains to my Bondi apartment, it took three days to re-open them.

My story was out there – and the shame was everywhere.

My declarations of dilation, sex and discovery were being listened to by everyone. The praise poured into my inbox, but I felt like it would have been easier to put a naked photo up on Facebook; I felt that exposed.

Was my need for social acceptance overtaking my healing? Was my ego overpowering my judgement? Was I trying to undo 18 years of fuck-ups in one bare-all announcement? This was an on–off cycle I often found myself in, which was the cue to stop, calm my buzzing adrenaline, and put some 'MRKH clothes back on'.

That's the thing about adjustment to a medical diagnosis. It can take years. As a successful journalist and author, Amy also understood the importance of taking stock of a public confessional. Even now, it's not uncommon for me to pitch Amy, as my mentor, an idea that is usually three months premature. Why? Because I can't always separate a wound from a scar, a sense of dread from excitement, a period of reflection from oversharing.

Today, the headlines don't bother me so much. In many ways, the reporters were right, I had been born without a vagina, but unlike when I first read those headlines, I no longer apologise for or scrutinise this honesty. This level of acceptance isn't for everyone, but as an advocate, I have always believed that if we only expose the fertility aspect of MRKH, we are telling only half the truth. A half-complete disclosure, for a half-complete body. If you are told for long enough that you are incomplete, you will believe exactly that: you are incomplete, less than, not enough.

We are living in a generation where hot-pink headlines on TikTok and Instagram are championing feminist rights. Where once bras were burned, advocates and activists are tearing up the internet with statements to quit body-shaming and eradicate online censorship. Social media exposure does not equal coping. We don't need to share all the facts before they are landed. We don't share our secrets, 'come out' to strangers and create a platform in order to 'fit in'.

Because, someone, somewhere, needs to see that breakages can be mended behind closed doors. For someone, somewhere, their today is my 20 years ago. For many people with MRKH, sitting in their bedrooms finding themselves creating a vagina, confused or ashamed, a headline means nothing. For those in corners of the world that are unforgiving of difference, your body isn't broken. And while I cannot get to everyone with MRKH, I hope my love can.

What does mean something is the way you feel in your skin today and every day. One accepting jigsaw of forgiveness at a time.

In fact, I want to ask every woman, 'How is your heart today?'

THIS TRAUMA WAS MEANT FOR ME

When we are in the midst of a trauma, the hardest words to hear can often be the most positive ones. For me, there are certain phrases that, even to this day, irk me: 'this too shall pass', 'look for the positives', and 'pain makes us stronger'. They might be true but they are, equally, massively unhelpful. When friends and loved ones rally to our recovery, bumper-sticker advice is the last thing we want to hear, aka toxic positivity.

Inwardly, I am screaming, 'But I don't want to be strong. I don't want to learn any more lessons. Just because I can be strong doesn't mean I want to be!'

And, exhale.

Recently, I was telling a friend how much I resist the word 'happy'. Not because I am not a fan of the word or the idea of people living with happiness, but because I don't know how to do 'happy' naturally. Every day, I wake up prepared to go into battle with a brain that edges towards being, sadly, sad.

For much of my life, even now, I look at my day and say to myself, 'What do you need to do today to bat for a better day?' Living with depression, or a past that is not easy to shake off, means learning to live with the fact that I am likely to always need a daily mental maintenance check.

I will always be someone who gets confused at people who say, 'I am of a bubbly nature.' My natural disposition towards sadness probably confuses them. I find positivity so scary, because it's not a place I visit often.

This is why depression remains so heavily misunderstood, because unless you walk in the shoes of a hopeless person, it can feel so unimaginable.

While I don't want to be identified as a womb-less woman, I don't want to be identified with the person who is always chatting about trauma. I don't want people to feel reluctant to answer the phone if they see my name calling. I don't want to be the person who is 'followed' by drama in other people's eyes.

In many ways, however, trauma is my specialist subject. Trauma, I know. Trauma, I can do. The most liberating thing I ever did for myself was to stop apologising for being sad. I decided to delete some phrases from my vocabulary, such as:

Sorry for disturbing you.

Sorry for unloading on you.

Sorry for sounding dramatic, or angry.

Sorry for being a blubbering mess.

Sorry for taking up so much of this conversation.

And weirdly, no one has ever put the phone down on me. No one has ever criticised my honesty. No one has ever unfriended me for not being chipper enough. So, why do we apologise for being human?

Perhaps by the end of this book, even chapter, I will discover why I have apologised for my past so much. Maybe, all along, this trauma was meant for me. Maybe your trauma, while hideous and harrowing, was pain you had to live through to tell a different story. Maybe your trauma was meant to be a soulful compass towards a different life, but only if you empower your trauma, instead of giving it free rein.

SEEING MY BODY THROUGH ADULT EYES

Strolling up Hall Street from Bondi Beach with salty hair and sandy feet was something I cherished after a day at the beach. I felt like I was living a life like a person who had 'made it'. I was barely earning enough money to cover my rent, but I really couldn't care less. What I wasn't buying in possessions, I was reaping in hope.

As the sun pitched down on my sun-kissed back, I was starting to feel like, perhaps, I was getting a second chance at life. I was learning what it was like to be single in Sydney, which I should state wasn't easy. I had no idea how to use dating apps. I didn't know the rules, the dating decorum or when was too soon to be head over heels for a guy.

I have to confess, I am one of those people who feel deeply, quickly. Not that you'd know it. After Tom and one brief encounter with a man on the edge of his nuptials, my 'play it cool' hat was anything but cool inside.

I was becoming a huge success in the world of women's advocacy and I was starting to awaken to my feelings around men, sex and intimacy. During one of the support groups in Sydney, the incredible psychologist (the same psychologist I met at a support group and walked out on as a teenager!) came to address us and I wanted to pull her aside to say thank you for the past, and thank you now for the present.

She remembered how incredibly angry I was. How much I despised my body, and the indifference I showed my diagnosis. I treated my vagina, infertility and subsequent trauma like they were nothing, although they were everything. As my eyes filled up with tears, she said, 'Ally, if there was a time in your life I would work over in therapy with you, it would be the time you spent in hospital undergoing vaginal dilation.'

The hospital was not at fault for this bad memory. Something in me was unleashed that day. The day where a nurse and trainee doctors circled my bed, as I pushed a tube into the entrance to my vagina. I was a child, lying on my back, being guided on how to push against the muscles where a womb should be sitting. A space where life should be growing. A space where love should be breaking. A body where a teenager should be living.

Even as an adult, I was ignoring this part of my past.

As a writer, I could write about my sexual organs, but I was unable to have sex without alcohol. As an advocate, I could talk about fertility, but I was unable to consider children in my future. As an adult, I was finding my way, but unwilling to go 'back there'.

While I was telling the story of my past, I was in the no-man's land between talking about my diagnosis and applying it to my present. And this would be the next stage of my story – and the hardest part to process.

Your sexuality is so much more than body parts. Safe sex is so much more than wearing a condom. Womanhood is so much more than being a mother. So, what would it all mean for me?

CHAPTER 12

The power couple of infertility

There's a saying, 'when something is right, it's easy'. I know this must sound like a massive generalisation, but for the first time, life made sense. I was (nearly) accustomed to reading about my '(wo)man-made vagina', my heart had healed from the break-up with Tom, and I was living on one of the most famous beaches in the world.

After a promotion at work, I had landed myself an office overlooking the Sydney skyline and was taking home a decent wage packet. While my corporate role didn't fill me with the same excitement MRKH advocacy did, I felt 'on top of my game'. My colleagues respected and admired me at the Sydney-based university and my work-hard reputation was getting me noticed.

Everything was falling into place. My parents would visit me in Australia at least once a year and, even though they probably wished their daughter was closer to home, they were proud of me for turning my life around. I had the job, the income, a healed heart, and my voice was becoming stronger.

Isn't that what any parent wants for their child? To be happy, free and successful in their definition of the word? I would often stare back at myself in window reflections in shock as I walked up George Street in Sydney.

I hardly recognised this well-groomed, power-suited, red-lipped women's health advocate. I went from an abused, bruised and exhausted pub landlady to someone who was starting to understand what peace felt like. What acceptance and hope felt like. What freedom and being alive felt like.

Now, if only I could maintain a healthy relationship ...

AN OVERNIGHT INSPIRATION

That's the thing about being an 'overnight inspiration' – everyone, including yourself, presumes you are cured. With every article, Facebook like, Instagram heart and TV appearance, I assumed that MRKH was a defunct part of my past and a reference to a happy present.

I couldn't, however, quite rest in my recovery.

Do you ever find yourself strutting down the road, listening to your favourite music playlist, and thinking, 'Yep, I am doing good. I like this life. How did this happen?' Don't think too hard about it, strut. Yep, you are nailing life!

It's in these moments when life feels too good to be true – cue, dread. If you've had trauma in your past, it can be hard to trust happiness in your present. Don't rock the boat on happiness, don't move too fast, because it might just disappear.

For people suffering depression, anxiety and trauma, life feels like a gentle mime show. Smile, but not too hard, because dread will hear you and fuck up the party. Date, but not too freely, because love will hear you and break another heart. Have sex, but not too soberly, because they may look back at you and find out the truth.

I was still navigating the world of dating apps, but only dancing around the edges and not committing. It seemed so ruthless and uninspiring, and like I was asking for trouble. The majority of stories we hear about dating apps and swiping our way to love usually ends in 'ghosting', 'breadcrumbing', 'submarining' and 'Marleying' (the contacting of an ex at Christmas ... yep, it's a thing!).

This was going to be a stage of my recovery that couldn't be fixed by raising my profile, appearing in a magazine or being interviewed on a podcast. I was still coasting pretty well on campaigning, beach time and yoga retreats, but I had no idea that I had my head in the sand when it came to love and partnering up in the future.

At the time, if you'd asked me about my ideal guy, I would have said someone creative, maybe a yogi; someone who would fit into my world. Instead, I was about to come face to face with a man who had spent his career staring at the part of a woman's anatomy that had tormented me for a lifetime.

Universe, are you laughing at me?

SORRY, DID THAT *REALLY* JUST HAPPEN?

In the April of my busiest year as an advocate, I flew to Queensland, further north than Sydney, for a conference. The event had been scheduled to launch and unveil a ground-breaking first for Australia. I knew it would rocket my profile as an advocate; I didn't realise it would trigger a secret relationship, which would almost be the breaking of me (again!).

When Doctor Greg entered the room, I was immediately in awe of him. The power that circulated around him was magnetic and everyone was poised for the moment when they could shake his hand, including me.

He was a highly sought-after expert in women's health. He travelled the world performing life-changing surgery, had a waiting list half a decade long and was at the forefront of an innovative treatment, which would open an incredible doorway for infertile women.

He also knew that he was special!

I remember how overpowering his energy was; nothing on earth could rattle or stun him. A camera crew from one of Australia's most popular news networks had been filming Doctor Greg's progress with a life-changing surgery that would help people like me, people born without a uterus.

I'll never forget the talk he gave, which was the main event of the conference. As the crowd took their seats and the studio lights and mics tuned in, I could see familiar faces around me. I recognised Australian doctors, nurses and MRKH patients that I had met on my campaign trail.

We all stared eagerly at Doctor Greg as he started to explain how he was one of the original surgeons to discover the procedure; a radical medical invention that could offer those who were infertile a chance to biologically carry a child. At this point, only a small number of live births had occurred through this procedure.

The operation was set to change the future narrative around infertility and I was sitting in a front-row seat for Australia's big reveal. At that time, I was terrified of public speaking, but I knew if I didn't speak up, I would miss my chance of being captured on camera and remain a stranger to the doctor too.

So, I did it. In a room full of TV presenters, cameras and hopeful mothers-to-be, I announced myself, my mission and described myself as a change-maker (I still don't know how I had the guts to do it!).

I'll skip the exact details of what happened next. Let's just say, a follow-up email led to an invitation to 'discuss my work' ... which led to a night of passion. The honesty in our sexual encounter was a revelation. I had introduced myself with my diagnosis and my condition, and he chose me. What's more, he kept choosing me again and again.

One minute I was dating random guys in Bondi, barely making it past the third date, and now here I was with my 'fertility hero'.

OK, our relationship had to be a secret to protect his reputation, but it felt very real with every interaction, every phone call into the night, every evening I spent at his hotel room when he was travelling for speaking engagements.

I became his confidante and I felt like I had a lot to offer because of – not despite – my past experiences. We would speak on the phone for hours every night, as he told me stories of how he treated thousands of women who became mothers following high-risk pregnancies. He seemed to idolise my tenacity and I idolised him. I was obsessed with him and I was sure it was love.

I remember telling Amy we were going to be the 'fertility power couple'. As a good friend, she did warn me that a secret relationship was likely to end in heartbreak, but the secrecy made sense to me. We weren't only protecting his reputation, we were protecting mine too. It helped me, having access to this amazing doctor who was at the forefront of innovation. People would think less of me if they knew I was sleeping my way into his attention. Wouldn't they?

My secret relationship was only shared with a trusted few. I didn't want to risk anyone discovering that I was dating a medical public figure; I didn't want to risk the trust that the community had put in me, that my care for them had an agenda. In fact, it had nothing to do with that.

With Doctor Greg, I could lean in to my diagnosis without any shame or fear of rejection. I didn't need to share anything about vaginal dilation or infertility grief, because he got it all. How was anyone going to match up to him? How was anyone ever going to set me as sexually free as he did?

I could even put up with our sporadic meetings. I knew, as a busy man, his time was scarce. To me, it didn't matter because I believed he wanted me. I would wait two weeks for a text back, a month for a phone call and a season to see him in person again. A year passed and I barely noticed, because my life felt fuller than it had ever been.

Our sex life was incredible. It was adventurous, experimental, and I was finding things out about my body that I had never known before. I was finding confidence in being touched in ways that made me feel like Anastasia Steele from a scene out of *Fifty Shades of Grey*. I know this may sound insanely cringe, but I was intoxicated by everything he exuded.

And, I am going to be honest, when you have a bad relationship with your vagina, and medical disclosures, it made complete sense to date a gynaecologist. He knew what he was getting into with more knowledge than any man on the planet. It was the extreme opposite of dating a man who joked about my diagnosis and then ignored it.

He saw me. The question was, did he really love me?

HOW THE MIGHTY FALL

The downside of dating a successful man is dating a successful man. After almost a year of our secret relationship, the limitations on my relationship with Doctor Greg began to feel like excuses. OK, you can't text me back because you're in surgery but what about the two days afterwards? I know you live out of hotels, but you do have a house – why do you never invite me to stay there? I know we both have reputations to look after, but what's the long game of this relationship – a lifetime of secrets and lies?

I was in a secret relationship with a global pioneer and I saw no way out or in. Unlike in our kinky sex life, there was no 'safe word' this time that was going to release me from the grip of this man. I did try to break up with him on many occasions. I tried to pull away, but I just felt so entangled.

For a sought-after surgeon with two PAs and a schedule planned a year in advance, he refused to prioritise times to see me. Our entire relationship was last-minute (which once felt spontaneous but now felt exhausting).

He would screenshot a flight ticket for the same day, and that was the only notice I received. Sometimes, he couldn't be bothered to get on the plane, despite me standing in the Sydney arrivals hall, eagerly waiting for him.

He never offered an apology and I didn't ask him for one.

Somehow, I had fallen into the same old pattern – shrinking to please another person. I was beginning to realise that my dreams of us being a power couple looked very one-sided – he was happy for me to do great things in my advocacy work, as long as it fitted with his ideas and his dreams (and his sex drive!).

One night, as I cried to Amy on the phone, I realised he had never suggested meeting my best friend. I was compartmentalising my life again, only this time it wasn't a diagnosis I was having to hide, it was the man I was in love with.

After one brief 60-minute encounter at 2 a.m. in a Brisbane hotel, I refused to kiss him goodbye. I didn't want him to leave, after such a short time together, mostly spent in bed. I was crying desperately as I begged him to stay a little longer. I hadn't seen him for two months. As always, he said he had places to be.

The night I refused to kiss him goodbye was the last time I ever saw him.

I wish I could say I was relieved, but I was heartbroken.

For three months, I would message, email and call him with no response. He didn't have social media, but he was still very much in the public eye. Once, I messaged his friend on Facebook to find some answers. I got nothing back.

He had vanished.

I hate to say this but it's true: I blamed myself. I was consumed with guilt that I didn't kiss him goodbye that day. I believed that it was my fault – that I lost a chance at love. It was my guilt that led me to stop eating, sleeping, smiling and hoping.

It took me two years to find peace with his early-morning departure out of my life. How I moved on isn't a 'quick-fix' story, but it is worth telling. Like every love story (or lust story), there are so many layers to the heartbreak. When I lost Doctor Greg, I not only lost a partner; I lost a dream of becoming a mother. Of course, I had hoped that he would 'cure' me too.

CHAPTER 13

What makes a mother?

It was a bumpy landing emerging from the relationship with the elusive doctor, but like any break-up, we find our way back. The dating carousel was getting tiring, and I felt like a failure as I reported to my friends that, yet again, 'it just didn't work out this time'.

Even with the Sisters for Love MRKH Foundation booming, I was starting to get a little embarrassed that I was the only one in the office, not just without a baby but without a partner. I was in the prime age for pregnancy announcements, maternity leave and baby showers. Even Amy had two children by now. Every Sunday, the group of people I could meet was shrinking as they gravitated towards the park and kids' birthday parties.

I remember skulking around the supermarket on a Friday night, with a cheap pizza, carton of juice and bar of chocolate. I felt pathetic and embarrassed. Sometimes, I would hide if I saw a friend or work colleague, fearing that they would twig that I was a sad little fuck-up!

I was terrified that my chances of having 2.4 children were becoming terrifyingly low.

My online community was thriving, but I was still putting the key in the door to a Bondi apartment with no one on the other side.

At this point, I was still being ghosted by Doctor Greg, months after the hotel goodbye that broke us. As a romantic at heart, I was unprepared to allow my experience with Doctor Greg to jade my perception of a happy ending.

So, I sluggishly downloaded Happn (my preferred dating app, as Tinder makes me *very* sad). I entered my name and bio, and uploaded a carefree and sassy profile pic. Again, I inserted my pre-loved profile description: 'ocean-loving, Shiraz-sipping, sandy-footed yogi'.

I had tried hiding my truth. I had tried radical transparency with the surgeon. Now, it was time to try somewhere in between. By now, I had more than enough in my baby fund to go through IVF and even get a surrogate (if I went to a country where this was legal).

But, did I really want to do it alone?

WAS THIS MY STAB AT MOTHERHOOD?

As the message appeared on my phone, 'Hey, Ally, nice to meet you,' I was back in the game! I had been matched with a hot Sydney photographer with a hip vibe about him. Luke was attractive, witty, charming and insanely down-to-earth.

Our first date was at a local bar down by Bondi Beach, and as I walked up to the front door, I remember thinking, 'If you can get over your former relationships then, Ally, you can do anything. Even a bad date.'

It wasn't a bad date. It was perfect. I jumped off my bar stool to greet him and I felt like I had known him for years. We instantly leant in for a kiss on the lips and smiled at one another, like we had both known this was going to be something special.

We talked for hours. We swapped stories of our days working in hospitality, how we had both overcome a troublesome past, and how we both loved trashy TV.

Then the question of all questions came: 'Do you want children?'

With a glass of wine, and first-date nerves, I made a beeline to the ladies' bathroom, slammed the toilet door and sobbed, saying, 'Fuck, I have to disclose again? What script should I use on this one?'

After I returned to Luke, I paused for what felt like an eternity. As I cleared my throat, I kicked off a turbo-charged conflict between truth and a chance at losing this guy.

In the MRKH community, disclosures of this nature are a BIG topic: how to tell a person you are dating that you are unable to carry biological children. Not only that, but with the MRKH disclosure, whether they google you or you reveal it first, the vagina part will be discovered.

It's hard to explain to young women the perfect scenario or perfect script, because it's different for everyone.

I would often consider several factors to assess if this is the right time and person to disclose to right now.

Do I trust them with a precious part of my story?

Why am I disclosing now?

Do I feel emotionally safe right now?

What's the purpose behind the disclosure?

Will it change the outcome of the situation right now?

Is my mental health stable today?

Am I prepared for the questions or reactions?

A mini self-assessment is key in these situations. As weird as it is, I have nailed my 'script'. I have edited, tweaked and rehearsed my script for years behind closed doors, so that when the words fall from my mouth, I'm not hearing them for the first time either.

'So, I am OK with what I am about to tell you. I welcome any questions that you may have, but you also don't need to say anything at all. I am telling you this now, because it feels like the right time in our conversation. When I was 16, I was diagnosed with a unique condition that I was born ... '

And this is where scripts can change.

#1: 'Without a uterus and vaginal canal,' for the days I feel ballsy.

#2: 'With an underdeveloped reproductive system,' for the days I don't feel ballsy.

#3: 'Without a uterus.'

Completed with ...

#1: 'I'm unable to carry children biologically, however, there're options such as surrogacy and adoption,' when I am undecided about motherhood.

#2: 'I'm unable to carry children biologically,' when I'm OK with being childless.

#3: Nothing. Disclosures are not an obligation on any level. We own our truth, on our terms and timings. I cannot stress this enough: we don't owe anyone an explanation, a permit, a licence or an acceptance plea.

I was lucky with Luke. I took option #1 and follow-up option #1, 'I was born without a uterus and a vaginal canal, and I'm unable to carry children biologically. However, there're options such as surrogacy and adoption.'

Not only was he accepting, but he was curious. I had barely got through the 'what' and the 'why' before he jumped in.

'Oh, right, so surrogacy is an option for you? Cool. I guess you don't have periods either. That's got to be a bonus.'

To me, this was the perfect response (although I can only speak for me, not the entire MRKH community). Luke said everything I needed to hear. Even though the absence of periods, sadly, validates my condition, if I am going to have MRKH, then I am not complaining about not bleeding monthly. While I craved a different script about womanhood and motherhood, in that moment, I could see Luke's desperate attempt to make me feel more comfortable.

THE NIGHT ENDED WITH A KISS

Months later, we were still happily dating. Like my last partner, he was a busy person, but this felt respectful and not full of excuses. When he was working late on a shoot, he would always check-in and tell me he missed me.

I was starting to feel the profound difference between being alone and loneliness, and the latter was no longer a reality for me.

I loved sitting in my apartment, squirrelling away with my foundation, sipping red wine, eating smelly cheese and thinking about this new man in my life.

I was creating a world where sex was softer (but great), dating was gentler, and perhaps I had a stab at a 'proper family' like everyone else. I may have been born without a womb, but I had been given an abundance of love. Infertility removes choice, but not every choice, and I was about to create my own ending.

I was starting to hear a sound that I hadn't heard before. It was my biological clock starting to chime.

Was this my chance at motherhood?

ON PAPER, I HAD EVERYTHING I NEEDED TO HAVE A BABY

On 8th January, I walked into an IVF clinic with Amy, who was by this time pregnant again. I was feeling an overwhelming surge of fear and hope. She had already conceived naturally multiple times, so we weren't there for her. I had an appointment to explore egg retrieval for the purpose of egg freezing.

I kept telling myself I was 'creating options'. However, it was much deeper than that – I was trying to explore how I *really* felt about motherhood.

It's a strange situation when, for your entire adult life, you've known that you're infertile but you're also not sure if you're even maternal. When, from the age of 16, you've been saving money for a surrogate but you're not entirely sure if you want children, even if you can have them.

The desperate search for clarity began.

As we left the clinic that day, another patient saw my weepy eyes and approached me sympathetically. 'It does get easier, I promise,' she said. She assumed the result I prayed for was a baby, when actually there was something I craved even more – clarity!

As an infertile woman, you are surrounded by sympathy from people who assume you'd do anything in your power to be a mother. When the clinic nurse read I was 37 years old, she asked, 'But why did you wait this long?' When I posted an article about motherhood on Facebook, a friend asked, 'Why would you post that ... in *your* situation?'

For 20 years, I have been aware that my body is incapable of having a baby naturally due to MRKH. On paper, I had everything I needed to continue my bloodline – a good egg count, enough money in the bank. I had even met a woman through the MRKH Foundation who was willing to act as my surrogate.

My potential surrogate was training to become a doctor and was passionate about the impact of infertility on women. Years before, we had connected through the MRKH medical network, and it felt like, well, destiny for both of us. We met, and discussed how surrogacy would work; the costs, obligations, boundaries and why we were the perfect womb-to-no-womb match.

I didn't tell Luke I was going to the appointment.

In my attempt not to scare him off, I kept this step a secret. While I pictured him sitting next to me at the doctor's office, holding my hand and listening intently to my medical results, a part of me knew that I was not the one for him. This was a part of my diagnosis even I was unprepared for. Struggling to process becoming a mother was daunting enough for me, let alone introducing fatherhood to a man who never expressed wanting to build a future for us together.

In the weeks following my appointment, I spent my time watching YouTube clips of women waking out of anaesthesia after the egg 'pick-up' procedure. I created an Excel spreadsheet and titled it 'Esme' – the name I would bestow on my daughter if I ever were to have one.

As an executive assistant at the time, I used my professional skills to plan a budget. I would see my $80,000 surrogacy fund decrease with every blood and hormonal result, transvaginal ultrasound and IVF clinic appointment billed by the Australian government.

I carried my scans, referral letters and results with me daily, as proof that I was taking on life independently. I was at the beginning of a new relationship with Luke and had told him about my condition. However, it was terrifying to break the news over dinner: 'I'm looking into freezing my eggs.'

I'm not sure if I was relieved or disappointed when he replied, 'That's a good idea ... for you and your future partner.'

As I don't menstruate in the typical terms, my IVF specialist wanted to wait a further six weeks before starting hormone treatment to boost and trigger my ovaries before egg retrieval, as he was a little unsure of the cycle pattern. That timeframe felt like an eternity but, as he said, 'You're in no rush – you don't even want a baby yet.'

Interestingly, that appointment was the one that made up my mind.

That evening, I went home and put my folder of admin in the bin. I was done. My IVF journey was over.

The hardest part was telling my surrogate that her gift should be given to a woman who was so sure. It was the toughest phone call I have ever had to make. I had it all – the funds, the specialists, the results and a borrowed womb – but I was saying, 'Thanks, but no thanks.'

Originally, I didn't regret my decision once. I realised, through the process, building a family with Esme was only an option if I was creating her with someone I loved and who loved me back. I know many incredible single parents, but it didn't, and still doesn't, feel right for me.

We do talk and she does know I love her, but I could simply not bring her into the world in the way I needed to. It was not my child's journey. Might I regret my decision not to freeze my eggs? Possibly. But I had to listen to my inner voice and, right now, all I feel is relief that I stopped forcing a path that was making me unhappy.

I'm so grateful I explored my parenting options, even if it was only to draw a line under them. Now, I know that a childless life is my choice and not Mother Nature's. I am no longer able to place blame on my body. I am infertile but I chose to be childless. And that's a powerful difference, even if I change it later. However, time is running out.

The only question mark was around Luke: what did this say about our relationship that I'd rather give up on my baby dreams than have an open and honest conversation with him?

PART FOUR

When will I feel like a woman?

CHAPTER 14

Female for a lifetime, but my year as a woman

When your current boyfriend refers to your future without them, the writing is pretty much on the wall. I chose to ignore the red flags with Luke; being his 'friend' and never his 'girlfriend', never meeting his family or friends, and the worst – overlooking a one-night stand after a casual confession by Luke. Despite Luke sleeping with other women and championing my egg-freezing plans ('for me and my future partner'!), that still wasn't enough for me to end things.

I forgave him. Or rather, I ignored the brutal truth that we were never going to work. That was until I found evidence that would ultimately end us.

Only three months after I discovered that Luke had been with another woman while I was in America presenting at a MRKH conference, I signed in to my iPad that Luke had borrowed.

As I sat in my office, I saw reams and reams of videos, messages and dating-app disclosures between Luke and other women. Every part of my body was shaking. These weren't messages from before his one-night stand, these were sexual exchanges from only weeks before.

It took me hours to scramble a text message together that read, 'I wish you had deleted your digital history, Luke.'

I didn't scream.

I didn't get angry.

I didn't cry.

I was eerily underplaying the impending break-up that I knew was coming for me.

That night, we had dinner together. Before I had even picked up my knife and fork to eat my pad Thai curry, Luke blurted out, 'You know I have never been in love with you. You must know this. You *must* know that I don't love you! So, Ally, it's over.'

Then we had sex, and I left.

For months, I would cry on a bench outside a local church on my way to work. In floods of tears, I would call my mum and try to understand why I wasn't enough for Luke. I took the brunt of his betrayal and I blamed myself, again.

It didn't matter if I had been on TV, national campaign, and world stages. The only 'like' I wanted on my Facebook feed was from him. My role as a public figure in women's health still wasn't enough. If fame and forgiveness weren't enough to secure a boyfriend, what more did I have to do to prove my 'enoughness'?

MY BABY, SHE DOES EXIST SOMEWHERE

One year after Luke and I broke up, I went to a baby shower that, in hindsight, I knew I shouldn't have gone to. Hiding behind sunglasses, my eyes were red and swollen. I was offering my congratulations, while painfully grieving my infertility. I can categorically say that I am not jealous of an expecting couple, but I am grieving for me. I can smile and mean every crease in my cheeks, but my heart can be aching simultaneously. It's a dual action that most infertile people will master over time.

I am not resentful, bitter or angry towards fertility. Every day, I think of Esme. Whether spiritual children are a 'woo-woo' concept or not, to me she does exist. It could be the storyteller in me that has to give her a name, from me, a mother who never quite got there. Either way, Esme has blue eyes, blonde hair, rosy pink cheeks, and a heart that will forever beat, somewhere out there.

I knew I always had the money in the bank in case I wanted to reconsider my decision.

However, I would later learn, last year in fact, that I would grieve her for a third time.

Sometimes, I feared that perhaps I didn't try hard enough for my dream baby. I feared that perhaps I wasn't willing to negotiate with the dream enough, because it didn't match my reality at the time. Perhaps, perhaps, perhaps ... I will always ask the questions with no solid answers.

After 42 years in an infertile body, did I give up a little *too* soon after all?

I didn't want to be a solo parent.

I didn't want to attend my baby's gender reveal standing alone.

I didn't want to be in a delivery room with no father to share the joy with.

I didn't want to be at an embryo transfer with my surrogate, as *just* one parent in happy tears.

I wanted the story. I wanted a family.

Emotional safety is everything, and that wasn't, isn't, part of my story.

If you are contemplating taking this path, prepare to prepare. The logistics, they are the easy bit, compared to the depth of your emotions, whatever the outcome. Gather support, be honest with the people around you, and give yourself permission to pause the process whenever you need to.

It's a biggie, and I wish you all the luck in the world when you go in search of your very own Esme.

Some heartaches can completely dismantle us. Whether it's a bad break-up from someone you loved who couldn't love you back, grieving a baby or infant loss, or an identity – some heartaches feel like they could kill you.

In just one year, I lost a boyfriend and a baby. I lost a future that I'd started to believe was my happy-ever-after ending. I couldn't explain my pain. I returned to the bathroom floor, contemplated returning to my old ways, and one night I nearly did.

I stared at the bathroom cabinet, with only a bottle of wine to keep me company. I was sobbing, mascara rolling down my face, dishevelled in my corporate suit and fearing that perhaps this time, I wouldn't make my way out.

I don't believe in entitlement – it's my biggest pet peeve in a person. I didn't feel entitled to a family or a husband, but I did question the big man up in the sky: God, why was love so hard for me?

What was the point in all the therapy, personal development, hundreds of hours on a yoga mat, Vipassana retreats, water cleanses, 'healthy friendships', if I was going to be back on that bathroom floor all over again?

Everything in me ached.

I would leave corporate events late at night to call a mental health line. I spent countless hours calling my mum to help me understand all the loss. I would threaten my future self with reviving my past self – because at least then, the pain made sense.

In fact, I was terrified. What if this was the heartache that would lead me to a drug addiction? It's not uncommon to have everything one minute and nothing the next. What if this type of grief, infertility grief and a broken heart, is too much pain for a bounce-back?

You can tell I was questioning everything.

Most of all, I was questioning myself as a woman more than ever. Boobs are one thing, but belief was another. A working vagina is helpful, but pleasure is another. Sex is nice, but desire is so much more. My XX chromosomal make-up recognises me as a biological female, but had I ever truly felt like a woman?

After a series of soulless one-night stands, my life no longer felt purposeful. My life as I knew it was coming to an expiry date – and only the global pandemic woke me up.

THE DAY THAT CHANGED THE WORLD

I am sure every writer authoring a memoir in the last few years will speak about COVID-19, the virus that stopped the world. I am no different. As global leaders shut down borders, authorities closed airports and economists halted the stock exchange, I took a frantic and scared phone call from home.

In total panic, my mum had heard the news that the Australian government was putting citizens on a 48-hour notice to return 'home'; travellers to leave, and those like me, in between two countries, make a choice and do it fast.

I knew she didn't mean it when she said, 'Ally, you have given so much to Australia, to your life and MRKH advocacy, but what will it take for you to pick your family?'

Geez. That was a punch to the heart.

But she was right. I had to make a choice and, after a sheepish request to my boss to work from 'home, the home 10,000 miles away', he kindly and effortlessly said, 'Yes.' I owe him so much for that moment because it was the decision that would change the next chapter of my life. Not only practical and professional choices, but choices that would force me to ask yet another big question: Ally, do you know your worth?

In just 24 hours, I locked up my apartment, handed over plant-watering duties to a neighbour and booked a flight to the UK. My aim was to return to Australia four weeks later, you know, to let the pandemic calm down for a few weeks. What a miscalculated choice that was!

Within hours, I knew life in the UK was going to be hard. Not only was it one of the hardest-hit countries, with the COVID-19 death toll reaching into the thousands daily, but also I had, like the world, access to nothing. No yoga, no therapist, no Amys, nothing. But I did have time and Wi-Fi, so what better way to put my boredom to good use than to hit the dating apps.

Despite loathing dating apps, it was the only connection I had with the local outside world. Within hours I had matched with a six-foot-three English hottie called Flynn. He was ripped, tanned (a plus considering the UK's climate), witty and too good to be true? Within days, I had already written the Facebook post in my head, outing our lockdown love story.

It was the ultimate rom-com story: a single woman returns from life overseas to take care of her elderly parents. At first, she struggles to settle back into a small English village, but then she meets HIM.

Of course, we abided by social restrictions. We exchanged countless messages, moved over to WhatsApp (because that's what you do when it gets 'real' #jokingnotjoking) and had a few Zoom dates. I would often text him, saying, 'Your Zoom room, or mine?'

I was seriously falling for this guy and once restrictions were lifted six weeks later, we met for a picnic by the river. I literally felt like I was in a movie scene; the water flowed, the birds tweeted, the sun bounced off his beautiful brown eyes, and he went in for the first kiss. There I was, soberly kissing this hot guy – this is it. I am home.

Weeks later, I was invited to his 'real' room for a sleepover. There's something really awkward about living back at home for the first time in years, and explaining that you 'won't be home' that night, aka, 'I am going to have sex with a man I met online.' We chatted and daydreamed the pandemic away.

We talked about if either of us wanted children, and we both agreed, we didn't. During one date, I found the courage to disclose my MRKH diagnosis. The words fell out of my mouth, and I only lost a few millimetres of sweat!

What he said next absolutely floored me. 'Ally, I know. I googled your name, your diagnosis, and I understand the best I can what you went through. I am not sure completely about the "vagina" part, but if penetrative sex isn't an option for you, that's OK. We can still do plenty of other stuff.'

For the first time in years, I had perfect, sober sex. For the first time in years, I had an orgasm, felt desired, felt immersed in pleasure, and didn't need a single glass of wine for it.

I was learning to be seen as desirable and valued. I felt confident and sexually empowered.

I also didn't have a choice but to commit to this life for now. Australia's borders were locked and, although I was an Australian citizen, I could only wait for a flight back, along with tens of thousands of stranded Australians.

After five failed attempts to return to Australia due to cancelled flights, and a government that had no intention of letting 'travellers' back in, I didn't care. This was the love story that I had been waiting for.

That was until, after stumbling upon (stalking) him on Facebook, I realised he had two children from a former relationship. We had talked about children and family, and he had never mentioned them. I couldn't understand the secrecy and I wasn't sure if I could handle being a step-mum to children who had been kept a secret from me for six months.

Despite being crushed, for the first time, I saw my worth. In one of our last conversations I said, 'It is not my job to convince you of my self-worth. It is not my job to be the truth teller for the both of us. I am worth more than secrets because I have worked too hard to unleash my own.'

At that moment, I picked myself up. For the very first time, I experienced self-love.

LET'S TALK ABOUT SEX FOR A MINUTE

During that break-up, I turned the biggest corner of them all. I knew I was 'Ally, the girl without the vagina', but I didn't know who 'Ally, the lover' was.

As you might have realised by now, I'm not a stranger to promiscuity, but sex still felt like something I did on autopilot. I had A LOT of sex in my twenties and thirties, despite being in two long-term relationships. Sex to me was ugly, like I felt I was. Sex to me was sordid, harmful, disrespectful and cheap. The way I had sex was the way I saw myself.

With James and Tom (Doctor Greg did not count), my only two long-term relationships, it became dutiful quite quickly. I experienced pleasure, but I didn't feel passion, because I didn't respect sex. I closed off my feelings and senses, like I had to when I first dilated. What it came down to was two body parts fitting – or not fitting – together. So, what if I changed the pieces of the jigsaw puzzle?

UNFEELING TO FEEL

Since my teenage years, I have explored bisexuality comfortably. I needed to be needed by men. I needed to know I was womanly enough for their advances. I also needed to be needed by women.

At times, I have deliberately pursued women, because they felt 'safer'. It would be fair to say that the contemplation of a relationship with a woman would give at least one of us the chance at childbirth. In essence, a long-term relationship could solve a pretty big problem.

Not that I would hand-pick a relationship because of fertility ... this isn't The Handmaid's Tale. But, somehow, an MRKH disclosure is so much easier with a woman; it's accepted and understood. In the few brief dating periods I have had with women, I have always felt confident, the dominant of the two. I have felt a masculine power emerge and it has felt natural to 'lead the way' in my same-sex interactions.

I have had some clumsy dates with women and some awkward sexual interactions. It turns out, learning about girl-on-girl sex from porn isn't very accurate. It was a steep learning curve at times. As I discovered, there's also etiquette in the gay community. I was pretty sure I wasn't doing 'it' right a lot of the time.

If you could see my leg jittering under the table as I type this, you'd know I am nervous about my sex life being scrutinised. I gave all my same-sex relationships a 'red-hot go', and I am so grateful to the beautiful women who showed me the way.

Like anyone exploring sexuality, it is complex, misunderstood and can trigger an entirely different set of confusing questions.

This is a totally important and necessary conversation, championed by the LGBTQI+ community, which I have so much respect for; communities that I have worked closely with during my MRKH advocacy work; and the powerhouse players who take a societal hit to normalise their life.

Let's hope that change, as incremental as it is, continues to break down the stigma. Little by little, we can light the flare that says difference is beautiful, and love is love.

FLIPPING MY PERSPECTIVE

We are getting to the pointy end of this book, where I am supposed to inject wisdom, insight, profound anecdotes and even solutions. I remain hopeful that the golden nuggets of my neurosis will emerge, but I am still not entirely sure how I can do the word 'woman' justice for you quite yet.

In fact, I am still recovering from talking about my sex life in such graphic detail, knowing that family members will either read this book or hear about it. I am not ashamed of my past, not now. When my pandemic love story dissolved and I eventually made my way back into Australia, I knew I wanted my future to look different.

I stayed in England for nearly a year during the pandemic, juggling my job in different time zones and waking up at 4 a.m. so I could speak to Amy while she gave her kids dinner. It was a strange time, living in two different worlds, still paying rent on an apartment in Bondi while living with my mum in a house we now co-owned (that's another story).

When I decided to return to Sydney, it was out of necessity. I couldn't keep hold of an apartment I wasn't living in. I needed to go back, at least for a while, to pack up my possessions and admit that the UK was my home for the foreseeable future.

The end of my relationship with Flynn was sealed when I told him I was leaving. Perhaps naively, I thought he would eventually fight for my return. Alas, all I got was a plane emoji after I told him I was Bondi-bound for the last time (at least for a little while anyway).

Unfortunately, re-entering Sydney meant 14 days of hotel quarantine, as Australia had some of the toughest COVID-19 restrictions in the world. As soon as I got off the plane, I was herded onto a coach and into the hotel room that would be my home for two weeks (at a cost to me of $3,000).

I wish I could say I sailed through hotel quarantine like some people, but I didn't. It triggered all of my emotional hurdles from the past, as I felt like I was trapped (which I was), alone (which I was) and all my choices had been taken away.

Every day, during my check-in with a mental health advisor (part of the quarantine programme!), I told them I was struggling and begged for them to let me out. At that point, the risk of COVID-19 was seen as more dangerous to the country than one woman's desperate pleas.

By the end of the 14 days, I was adamant I was not going to stay in this country, which had just constrained me.

Anger can be quite the motivator, I found. I was so angry that my pleas for mental health support were going unheard, as policemen with guns would guard the doors to our rooms. I used this anger to fuel me back to a life in the UK. I knew I had changed while in the UK and I feared the consequences of living in a country that could so strategically and cruelly keep families apart. Not even death was a good enough reason to allow a person to leave or enter the country.

While in the UK, I discovered that Bondi has a shelf-life. Few leave the 'Bondi Bubble' because it's a special, special place. For those who do, they will often say that love leads them away. Love for themselves, another person, a new career or a venture was the pull to leave the majestic waters of the Eastern Suburbs.

The day I handed in my notice at the job that had given me a chunky income, a safe schedule, lifelong friends and a ten-year excuse for not aiming higher was a scary and liberating one.

It was one of the hardest decisions I had to make, to leave my best friends, my favourite yoga studio and a life that had once saved me. For the first time in my life, I was ready to take myself out of steadiness. I was hungry for a new life, in this new body, with new self-worth, because my self-worth was steady in me.

CHAPTER 15

Can truth be trendy?

One of the most pivotal points in my storytelling journey began with Amy and me standing in her kitchen, sticking my old dilators into different types of fruit to see which best resembled a vagina on camera. It is testament to our friendship how seriously Amy took her role as creative director. She knew the end result wasn't just an Instagram reel – it was a huge step in 'outing' my deepest secret.

Despite a lot of MRKH sufferers documenting their journey online, at that time, I had never seen anyone openly talking about 'the process' – how the 'fix' really took place. We have been conditioned not to talk about that bit – the pain, the process, the indignity, the 'white-knuckling' or creating your own vagina where there isn't one naturally.

I had a week before I left Australia to move home to the UK for an indefinite period. Before I left, I had arranged to stay with Amy and her family for a week, to say goodbye to the kids who, in a way, felt like my own.

As I packed my bag for my stay at Amy's, I decided to cram in one last item – my vaginal dilation kit. I have always had a kit close by just in case I needed to add a 'little' length in the absence of sex.

Amy's husband was used to our creative collaborations. He didn't bat an eyelid as he watched us set up her tripod. With half a melon and a kit of dilators, we told the story of what women, if diagnosed with MRKH or a similar condition causing the vagina to shrink, tighten and lose length, will ultimately face. Four weeks later, this video had been viewed over 429,000 times.

As I saw the number of Instagram plays creep up to the thousands, as an MRKH advocate and charity leader, I was thrilled. Over 21 peer groups and charities exist globally to offer support and raise awareness of this unique condition, and this 30-second video was being viewed by onlookers internationally.

As we packed up the tripod and ate our rock melon prop for breakfast, my oversharer's nerves set in. Had I gone too far? Did I edge too close to the topic of vaginas? My vulnerability hangover, however, was matched with pride. As my comments feed and DMs started to fill up with messages from doctors, hopeful mums and people with MRKH, I knew something special was happening.

In just 30 seconds, I had rallied a global narrative.

That reel would have an incredible ripple effect, leading to interview requests from major publications across the world and uncountable emails from women with MRKH saying thank you; thank you for telling the reality of our condition.

What I didn't see coming was the impact on my relationship with my charity.

A year earlier, the Sisters for Love MRKH Foundation had rebranded its digital doors, to create a bigger, broader and internationally recognised hub within Australia.

Prior to leaving Australia, I had informed the charity that my role and responsibilities would remain the same. After all, we were emerging from a global pandemic, where working from anywhere was the new norm.

It was a role that saved me in many ways, despite it also saving others. I felt proud of the work I had achieved, and some of my closest friends are those who joined me on this journey. Unfortunately, some people – not all, but some – within the organisation believe the story I shared should have been kept behind closed doors.

TRUTH MIGHT COST YOU, THAT'S OK TOO

For much of my life, many of my 'truths' have felt lodged in the back of my throat like a stuck chicken bone. Much like a bad dream, where you struggle to run, talk or walk and, despite every effort, you're trapped in nightmarish quicksand. It's like I had 'soul paralysis'. I kept making every effort to share my thoughts, feelings, fears and needs, yet the words felt impossible to part with.

We believe freedom is gained in the control of what we say or do not say. Of course, some truths are ours to hold on to. I've never felt the need to share my vagina monologue with colleagues around the water-cooler. Not every lover needs to know my backstory and not every interview requires me to spill my guts.

I've also shared the odd lie when it feels easier than telling the truth. There have been times I've not wanted to make people feel uncomfortable by sharing my vagina story. Do people really want to know about MRKH? Are they really curious about it or would they prefer I stop talking about my "things down there"? Reading the room is difficult, and it's hard to know just how polite to be with your trauma. Sometimes, it's perhaps easier to forgo your own truth for the sake of sparing others' discomfort. When half-truths and fibs come easily, it's not necessarily deceitful or even intentional, it's maybe just because the truth is a little too hard.

Downplaying a truth has always come quite naturally to me, which is a dangerous personality trait. Like the time I learnt that Luke was unfaithful and proceeded to eat my spaghetti bolognese as if nothing was wrong.

By handing out confident lies and staying composed in emotional chaos, I was withholding my truths. The only problem with this theory

– that thinking a lie or silence is better than freedom – is that an unspoken truth can turn toxic.

When the email from the charity landed with a clang in my inbox, expressing their unease at my reel, I had two choices: backtrack, apologise and try to undo the exposure; or stand by my truth and my belief that this story mattered.

It was brought to my attention that 'several' members of the MRKH community were 'triggered' after seeing me reshare an article about my reel on a respected Australian charity's social media platforms.

There have been many decisions in my life I've grown to question, but this wasn't one of them. I was, of course, sorry that the article had triggered a number of people, but this number was in the minority.

Since the article was published, I'd received an overwhelming response from advocacy leaders in the LGBTQI+ community, patients, parents, doctors and others in support of this article.

I believed that, by withholding the story from the MRKH community, we would further add to the culture of shame that people with MRKH face. By deleting our story, we were at risk of sending out the message that dilation is something to be hidden and that the reality of our condition should be a secret.

This was a chance to have an honest, open and empowering conversation with our community. I truly believe that part of our duty is to address the triggers and not remove the source of them.

I stated all this when replying to the email.

I wish I could say I rallied at the injustice, but I shrank with shame and embarrassment. I felt like I was 16 all over again. In retrospect, I can see, it hit me at a time when I was already vulnerable – packing up my life in Australia and starting over (again) in England.

This is the part they don't warn you about when sharing your truth – not everyone will support the exposure. Do I regret it? Not today. I do concede that, in retrospect, the social media post could have included a 'trigger warning'. I do not believe it was inappropriate to share. In fact, I hope it creates a ripple effect of truth-telling across the community.

At the time, I thought I was grieving the end of my relationship with the charity. Now, I can see, my sadness was hiding anger. This shame is the reason people never recover. This backlash is the reason we hide in the shadows. This reaction is the reason that so many women, like me, never feel they can tell the world, 'This is me.'

I might not be a mother, but I want to teach our children, and our children's children, that speaking our truth can be the coolest, hippest and trendiest act of self-love. So, when I returned to the UK, with 19 boxes and my IVF nest egg sitting in the bank, I was determined that this time round, I was going to take England by the balls!

I NEEDED A NEW STORY

As my lockdown love story with Fynn didn't go according to plan, I was young (ish), free (living in my childhood bedroom) and single (#holyshit). I had the perfect plan. If Elizabeth Gilbert can become a bestselling author by eating pasta, praying and falling in love, so could I.

Admittedly, I didn't have a plan, but for the first time in my life, I was 100 per cent free to live out my overdue 'gap year'. I was going to travel, write, find myself a handsome local in a little Greek fishing village and be free.

There is a famous phrase that I need to share with you. It's also worthwhile if, like me, you are a strategist for your future to note down for whenever life goes a little tits-up.

If you want to give God a laugh, tell him your plans.

Returning to your home country doesn't mean you are returning home. For 15 years, I had been a visitor at my family's home, and a tourist in my village. I would recognise the odd familiar face but in essence I was a stranger. I realised pretty quickly that I was in for a bumpy landing. I had travelled 36 times between Australia and England. Jumping on a plane for me was easier than finding a bus route. I knew Changi Airport in Singapore so well I even made a dating-app connection there, whom I still chat with as friends. I convinced myself that the transition would be easy; after all, I was back home.

Naive, Ally.

With flights still grounded following the pandemic, the prospect of my Greek-god holiday romance was dwindling by the hour. I didn't feel creative. I didn't feel free. I felt scared.

I love my parents, but for most of my adult life I had lived in a different country to them. I had funded and fought for my independence. For nights, I would stare at my ceiling recognising the same grooves along the skirting board that were there when I was 16 years old. I was lying in the bed where years before I had made my vagina.

My European-based friend, Emily, who I had met years earlier at YogaBliss, assured me that everything I was feeling was 'normal'. She had moved to Europe after she fell in love with her husband. But I hadn't fallen in love. I had no one. A few boxes, no job, and I was left wondering, 'What the fuck have you done?'

It didn't make sense to me. I loved my parents, and their pure glee at seeing me daily moved me to tears too. I saw such potential in my future in England, but I felt like I had lost everything that saved me.

No yoga, no friends, no structure and no fucking plan.

It became glaringly obvious one morning that I wasn't here to find my 'Eat, Pray, Love' year, I was here to discover my mum's. I had saved my past, and now it was time to save hers.

EVERY STORY HAS A PLOT TWIST

Eleven weeks after I landed in England, I held my dad's hand and said, 'But, I'm not ready!'

After returning home from a morning stroll, I had found our back gate ajar and an ambulance parked outside. It was one of those dreamlike moments, where your legs move slowly, your eyes gaze for the trauma target, and your heart stops beating.

Lying on the floor, contorted and unconscious, was my mum, surrounded by paramedics and beeping machines.

I rushed to her side, stroked her exposed belly in circular motion and repeated, 'It's OK, Mum, it's going to be OK.'

I have never feared death or misunderstood God as much as I did in that moment. As we stepped out of the ambulance, I was told to wait outside. I was choking on the shock. I called my dad, who lived close to the Berkshire hospital. My mum's partner at the time was already enroute.

Within hours, my mama was admitted to ICU following a series of after-shock seizures, due to her stroke eight years before. There was no explanation or conclusion, other than 'these things happen'.

I remember leaning over her, as tubes hijacked her frail frame, and whispered with salty tears, 'Please, Mum, please wake up.' I begged her to wake up. I pleaded against her forehead to wake up. I needed to call my mum, to tell her how scared I was. I needed her, to help me help her.

We waited days and days, where COVID-19 restrictions gave us just 20 minutes by her bedside each day. The morning they told us that they would attempt to wake her up – the make-or-break moment – I have never prayed so hard. I have never promised God so much.

The hospital corridor was so quiet and I have never felt so alone. At first, I wasn't sure if I could watch the tubes being removed. I didn't know if I could wait seconds to see her eyes flicker open.

Then, her eyes flickered. Disorientated, she scanned the room, needing an explanation. She was confused, traumatised, and seemed so, so small.

As I type this, it's the first time I have re-lived this moment. Tears are fogging up my glasses and I need to finish this chapter, so I can go and hold my mum again.

Because she did wake up – in more ways than one. Her re-entrance into life was the boldest it's ever been.

I'm not going to sugar-coat her recovery – the early days back at home were hard. Brain trauma is one of the biggest traumas a body can overcome. Gradually, she found her steadiness and peace. Suddenly, she found her truth. It was time for her to live differently.

Within four weeks, her 25-year relationship was over.

Overnight, my purpose became supporting my mum through her greatest transition. Over an eight-month legal battle, we raised the money to buy her ex-partner out of the house. Part of this money was my IVF fund – Esme's entrance ticket to the world.

As I transferred the final dollar into the solicitor's bank account, I sat against my bedroom radiator, sobbing for Esme. I couldn't comprehend that she was really gone, this time for good.

My mum knew why I'd been saving that money all these years. There were many nights when I cried and she apologised, but neither of us undid the decision.

I knew we needed to keep our home. My mum and I needed a future back together again. We had spent years bouncing between countries, break-ups, traumas and revelations.

We bought back our home and we bought back our future.

In the back of mind, despite previous doubts, I've always thought the next stage of my life would involve becoming a mother. In fact, it was mothering my own mother – and what an honour it is.

MY GOODBYE

Infertility grief continues to flip my perspective on a daily basis.

It is never truly curable, the loss of motherhood. So many – too many – people are grieving quietly. Staggeringly, 1 in 8 people experience infertility and 1 in 4 experience miscarriage or infant loss. Yet, women and men are swaying quietly in their homes, wondering if they will ever meet their Esme.

One night, I wrote these words and sent them to Amy, who cried along with me. You forget the ripple effect of infertility. While apologising, Amy admitted she also grieved my infertility – two best friends who would never feel the bond of raising babies together. These are the kinds of truths we need to speak about – the ones we can't fix, which still need to be spoken to be freed.

To you, my final goodbye,

Esme, you have blonde locks of hair, sparkly ocean-coloured eyes, and a grin that could break a million hearts. Your giggle is gentle and mischievous. You have the cutest, chubbiest thighs that I want to sink my teeth into daily.

Esme, you smell like marshmallows and bubble baths.

You fall asleep to me singing the lullabies I once fell asleep to.

If I allow my gaze to fixate on a window long enough – a moving tree, or wisp of air – I take it as my sign that you are gently saying, 'Mama, I know you wanted me there.' And I am. In the space where my womb would sit, where your heart is thinking of me, I am here.

Please don't stay blurred for too long, because I am desperate to see all of you.

Please be happy and safe.

Please wait for me.

You will always be mine.

Love always,

Your mama

It's amazing how opening up space in your life allows newness to enter your orbit. I felt as though my identity had disintegrated, as I shed so much. If I wasn't going to become a mother, digital nomad or charity leader, who was I going to become?

But then I met him.

CHAPTER 16

Have I qualified as a woman?

While I was living at my mum's house – now 'our' house as I was officially co-owner – I developed a new addiction: googling. I'm not referring to 'What are the best shows on Netflix?', or 'What is the joint net worth of the *Real Housewives of Beverly Hills* cast?' Well, that's a lie, I do that a *little* bit too.

I am talking about the real-life curiosities that only the internet can apparently solve: 'How long in a relationship before you are officially a couple?' 'What attachment style am I?' ('Anxious' apparently; thank you, Goop!) 'Does he miss me too?' This is the way we live nowadays – distrust the gut, trust the internet.

When I admitted it to my friend Susie, we both laughed, because it was funny. Funny because at 41 years old, I need validation via an algorithm. Funny that I wasn't asking myself first. Funny because, even after years of therapy and self-help work, I wasn't asking the person who could tell me the answers I craved: him.

'Him' was a new guy. A guy with an amazing story of his own. Our relationship had started out as a friendship, as a result of internet scrolling (see, it works sometimes!).

One day, I was searching for an Instagram account where I could share my story about self-harm and recovery. A beautiful friend, poet and artist, CeCe, pointed me to a social media site where I could potentially share the story behind my scars.

As I scrolled through their feed, reading captions written by brave storytellers, there was one story that had me hooked – Jack's.

Jack was a man who had overcome cancer – a very unusual kind of cancer for a man. He was honest, accessible, courageous and real. Among a grid of female faces, I was in awe of this one lone man, standing proudly behind his past.

I wasn't looking for romance or a digital flirting partner, but I knew I had to reach out to him.

Within days, we were on video calls for hours.

He told me his story and I told him mine. Oddly, or brilliantly, I didn't think twice before delving into my 'vagina tales', and how my medical diagnosis set me on a path, like his cancer diagnosis did for him, towards freedom and awareness work.

Off and on, we would exchange messages, voice notes and pep talks on difficult days. I would offer him dating advice, and likewise, he did back. It felt freeing and easy to be talking with a man so honestly. I wasn't hoping he would fall in love with me, accept me, date me, and certainly not have sex with me. For the first time in my life, I was in the most honest friendship with a man.

I was so proud of him, and even more so, proud of me. I didn't need to have sex with a man for love and respect. It was a friendship like I'd never experienced before.

MAGIC!

As I walked away from Jack after our first in-person coffee hang, I knew he was special. I had been back in England a couple of months at this point and this was my first 'proper' day out since my mum had became unwell. We wandered the streets of Oxford, and I found myself fixing my hair and sneakily applying some lipstick. I suddenly realised, I wanted Jack to fancy me.

Nothing happened that day between us, but when I left him, I knew that this was the kind of man I wanted to date. My dilemma brain soon kicked in, as I wondered, 'What would happen if our friendship was replaced by sex and fear? Would the friendship vanish?'

Two months later, I was on a train to see him again. I was still saying to my mum (because we are *that* close), 'Nothing is going to happen, we are good friends and that's perfectly enough.' The only thing was, I was wearing new underwear, on the off-chance (hope) that he would make a move.

We are still undecided who made the first move (because, sexy egos!), but for the next two days after that night, I was ridiculously giddy. As we said 'goodbye' at the train station, I was too coy to turn around and wave at him, despite him waiting for me to do so.

I just knew that this was something incredible, and I couldn't believe how unexpected this man was.

How was this happening to me?

Every day, we would talk for hours. With 200 miles between us, and fortunately as great communicators, our conversations were tender, sensitive, flirty and certain. I felt so safe with him: physically, emotionally and sexually.

Our months of previous friendship had secured our trust. I knew how he dated women, how he approached difficult days, how he cried and how he laughed. The 'getting to know each other' was done.

We had all of that and then we had magic on top. He is both my best friend and my lover.

One evening, he took me to a book launch for one of my favourite authors. As she told her story of recurrent miscarriage and the palpable pain of fertility struggles, Jack took my hand. He tenderly placed his palm around mine, because he knew that I would be triggered. Even though I was hanging off every word the author said, my eyes started to water.

I was desperately trying to avoid a public meltdown, and then the penny dropped: perhaps every heartbreak before this moment had led me to him.

The fact that we are both advocates for stigmatised and taboo medical diagnoses makes this romance almost too good to be true. We talk about the day our lives changed because of what a doctor reported to us. We talk about how our past relationships broke us, and then how we rebuilt our worth back together again. There is chemistry, there is respect and ... there is a lot of fear.

Cue Google.

This is the part where I am not sure if I am jinxing my future with an 'honesty tattoo' by talking about it so hopefully.

I have no idea what our future holds. With his life in the North of England, and mine in the South, the days I miss him often override the fondness. We thrive on independence, so the set-up currently works, but the biggest and scariest part isn't thinking, 'When am I going to see him again?' It's how my heart feels when I leave.

Now I can see where I have healed and the steps it takes to get there. Opening myself up to such a love is fucking terrifying but I know now that I'm ready for some types of love, to bring me back to life.

I don't know what will happen an hour, week, month or year from now. What I do know at this moment is that men like Jack exist. I am forever grateful to him for exposing me to this gentle, honest, rare type of love. His story is brave and so is he. Men like Jack need to be held tightly, and while I have no idea how this story will end, I am so grateful that he is part of mine today.

Because every day, I am learning how to love differently. I am learning how to love with trust and not to mistake silence for betrayal, or anger for harm. And I'm learning, finally, that I am worthy of real love.

BOUNCING BACK IN A BIG WAY!

There is something to be said for fear – the good kind of fear. The fear that reminds us that we are alive and healing enough to feel it. For the first time in my life, I am not scared of the future.

I get concerned when things don't go my way or when Jack and I have an argument. I fear seeing my parents age, and that one day I won't see my mum's big blue eyes smiling at me each morning. I fear that my story can't just be about 'vaginas and trauma', and I fear that I'll have no other 'wow' story to tell.

I fear that I will not overcome infertility grief and I fear that with every year, the space around me will grow. I fear that I will never get these words published, despite this book being a dream for the last ten years. I fear that my closest friends will forget about me, as they continue their lives in every country but the one I am in.

Don't worry, there is a point to my fear list.

Despite the fear, there is hope.

Even when I am unable to predict – and trust me, as a Taurean I like to predict – I know that I will always bounce back. I am someone who openly owns my depression. I take a pill every night at 7 p.m. to balance out what my brain cannot. This pill may be in my life forever or, one day, I may stop taking it. I am content and accepting either way.

No longer do I need to stand behind a charity to tell my story. I don't need to make love drunkenly in the dark, because I know that my body is worthy. I am not longing for the day that my life will start, because today, I am in the yummy thickness of my own story. And finally, I trust myself to make good decisions.

Here is one of them.

I sent Amy a picture of my boob. It was a vulnerability exchange after she sent me a picture of her naked body on the beach. She was in a full handstand, with her blonde hair scraping the sand, with her beautiful vulva on show. Man, I zoomed in and thought, 'Wow, she's beautiful, but I could *never* do that with another woman.'

I often joke with Amy that she has always been six months ahead of me in the self-love club. So, while I didn't send her a picture of my own vulva, at 6 a.m. a photograph of my tanned, gravity-tortured boobs landed in her inbox.

Fuck it.

This moment of brazen boob bravery was my message to her, and to me, that I was no longer battling with my body. In the comfort of a safe exchange, it was my way of saying, 'Look at me!'

Like a best friend should, she sent me back a dozen 'flames'. With my consent, she also showed it to her husband, because she was so proud of my progress. As part of my inner circle, she knew this wasn't just about a nude selfie – it was a badge of honour for the life I'd survived and a reclaiming of myself.

This isn't my nudge for you to get your boobs and vulvas out and start snapping pics (we all know the dangers of cyber insecurity!). However, in the comfort of your home and body, feel it, touch it, get curious with your curves. Discover your pleasure points and what makes your skin go 'goosey'.

This might feel a bit weird, and that's OK too, but maybe one day, give this a go:

Make love with you.
Climax with you.
Lie naked with you.
Honour you.

Forgive your body for not always working.
Forgive your genes for mutating.
Stroke the creases around your belly and boobs.
Close your eyelids and fantasise.
Fantasise about desire, pleasure and power.
Hold your scars and thank them for healing.
Hold your hips and thank them for curving.
Hover your fingertips above your heart, and say thank you for loving.
Circle your womb space and say thank you for feeling and healing, for what it may or may not have grown here.

I don't have the magic formula for finding inner peace, acceptance and self-love. But, lovely, please, if you are in pain, please stop. Please, please stop. Believe that there is a different story in your book. There is a different chapter where you can find hope, love and liberation.

I wish I could squeeze you right now. Maybe one day I will. Maybe one day we will be friends and be shoulder to shoulder, happy together.

Until that day, I know there is a brave, bold, beautiful, lumpy, bumpy, imperfect human behind the hands that are holding this book.

WHAT IS A WOMAN?

Never has my knee twitched under a table like it is now as I get to the end of this book. Isn't this the part of the story where I reveal the operatic conclusion? Am I supposed to find society's answers to womanhood? Will I reach the crescendo behind the stigmas that continue to haunt the infertile? Are vaginas at the epicentre of what qualifies us to be a woman? Or, am I going to keep throwing rhetorical questions out there, in the hope that the answer will land with you?

OK.

Here goes.

In my eyes, womanhood is fiercely complex and yet massively simple. One answer comes from the opinion of people you do not know, and the other comes from you. For years, women have been educators, academics, nurturers, teachers, mothers, boardroom bad-asses, wives, lovers, carers, leaders, childless, childfree, gurus, followers, baby-making-machines, walking vaginas and females.

We know, however, this is not always the case in everyone's eyes.

Not all women bleed, and many men do.

The gender conversation is rife, necessary, misunderstood and accepted. Society, if you cannot tell, questions, 'What qualifies a woman as a woman?' We have become a walking contradiction. We have become, dangerously and sadly, a society both progressive and regressive in our debates. In our society, we see so much change, and in parts of the world, we see none.

We see honour killings inflicted on those with MRKH by the shame this choiceless diagnosis brings. The MRKH community sends vaginal dilation kits to women in developing countries, because they are forbidden under their own rulers to receive them locally. My life 20 years ago is someone else's today. It's a lonely, staunch and cripplingly taboo place to exist.

We have made so much change and prompted the conversations that matter. However, we can and must do more.

In one breath, women have a choice and, in the next, a senate is choosing the rights of a woman's body. The rising and terrifying stats of domestic violence cases against women continues, and yet, social media has never been more capable of campaining for change on a global level.

So, so many people struggle due to how they perceive their bodies.

Whether it's through eating disorders, abuse, self-harm or medicine, there are people, like me, who have spent decades in a body they loathed and blamed for not working. There is nothing more painful than living in skin that you feel unwelcome in. For all those who are battling depression, danger, sadness, recovery and treatment: I hear you, I see you. And I only have love for you.

I must also say that while this book is about my journey and perceptions around womanhood, there are men out there with the same tears, fears, pains and traumas that I have experienced. Let's not forget them. Let's not forget that every being on this planet deserves love, compassion and an opportunity to be heard equally.

MY ANSWER

Throughout this book, you may or may not have noticed that there is one word I've never used when referring to myself: a woman.

Not once have I called myself 'a woman'.

This was a conscious and deliberate decision, because I wanted to determine through writing this book if I would ever find the answer to the question that has haunted me my entire life: 'When will I feel like a woman?'

> My answer is, I have always been a woman.
> However,
> My love for me got lost in the chaos.
> My love for me got hidden in the numbness.
> My love for me was buried in the trauma.
> So I asked, 'What would love do?'
> Love would want me to be happy and free.
> So, Ally, you've arrived at love.
> Ally, you are a woman.

Something didn't sit right with me after I wrote the above and slept on this chapter for a few nights. Every part of me wanted to deliver the ultimate ending, that I had all the answers and I was a loud, proud and roaring woman. However, this wouldn't be true.

That's why I left my words, but struck them through for you to read.

Every day, my perception of my own version of womanhood changes. I have big boobs, that's never changed. I know I can hold babies, and have a loving, sexually safe relationship.

So, what's left? Choice? Freedom? Acceptance?

I know I have those.

I can't say I have arrived at the big 'definition', because the truth is, I don't know if there is one. I don't think there is an answer, just a feeling.

What I do know is that I have and will always be in pursuit of a better day. I do know that I want to live my life with kindness and compassion for myself and others.

Today, I like being me.

Today, I am happy and that's plenty.

So, go gently.

Big love,

Ally xo

Epilogue

It has been over 12 months since I wrote the final words in Chapter 16. So much has changed since then. So much that has taught me about kindness, love, purpose and persistence. Shifts in key relationships, which have taught me about grief, discovery and self-belief, and about my ability to trust my worth. Perhaps my cockiness that MRKH was the last batch of pain for me was a tad naive and clumsy. Because life has demanded yet more surrender, more softness, and further subtle recovery.

Today I am heading to London, back to the hospital where my story began. Unlike 26 years ago, today my purpose is very different. For nearly four years, I have been the 'designated safe person' for a young woman with MRKH.

Today, I've arranged to meet her at the hospital as she starts her journey with dilation. I feel a good-kind-of-weird. On the one hand, I am going back to the scene of my "trauma crime" and on the other, I have never felt more ready to move on with my story.

The fact that she asked me to come is an honour. It seems such a long time since I was lying on that hospital bed. I wish I'd had a 'me' back then. So, that's my plan today. I will follow her lead, hold her hand and give her the permission to think that none of this is meant to feel OK. I will take her for lunch and try to make her smile. I will acknowledge the tears. I will show her that there can be a safer way to live, when nothing feels sure.

These three days in hospital don't have to become her trauma story. So, I will walk through the hospital entrance, and put my ghosts to rest. I will not replay the looping image of me lying on my back, alone, creating a vagina. I am tired of being a hostage to my past. I want to be Ally, without the four letters MRKH.

Unexpectedly, there are people in my book who played an important part in my life, who are no longer part of my story today.

Amy and I once discussed how much of our past needs to remain there. We chatted about how to revamp our stories to grow with us and not become the only story we have. I never want to be the cover band who plays to an empty pub because my life is out-dated and not special or relevant anymore.

I am learning that legacies are not all they are measured up to be. However, I love speaking to the press, booking a podcast and carving out my next collab. My 'healthy' addiction of choice is creating projects that only a national and international platform is fit for. I'll admit it, I am fine with a bit of friendly fame. While I like money, I like people more. I need my life to make sense, because why else did all the hurt happen if it's not to shape the ways we can heal better?

In the absence of offspring, I have always panicked that I need to do more. I need to fill in the time where the children would have been. If I am not a wife or a mother, then what's my claim to a successful life? Like my ambitious circle of friends, we are all waiting for that next big 'wow' moment, like an excited surfer catching a mountainous wave.

Regardless of who you are, what role you work in, or how you define your purpose, legacies are great, but happiness is better. A win can be getting up in the morning, after a week in a hole. A red-carpet moment can be watching a movie, holding the hand of someone you thought you'd never meet. A big career break could be just that, a break from your career to study your lifelong passion in filmmaking or floristry.

My friends are survivors, storytellers and people who remain loyal to their past, if it means helping someone else combat their present. However, there is something in me longing for something different. I want to be more than my diagnosis.

I want to trust that there is still a different story in me.

I *wanted* to trust that my movie ending was a happily-ever-after with Jack. It was not.

I want to trust that this book will help you in the ways you need.

The most important thing I have learnt, and am still learning, is to surround yourself with people who have a desire to love you. Surround yourself with people you want to love. Tell yourself that you too are worthy of a real love. This may mean making some difficult choices, as I have had to recently, but you and I are worth it.

This morning, as I held my mum's hand while she battles with her health, I smelt her hair for a little longer than usual. I need to remember that she made, saved and has loved every inch of me. I texted my dad to tell him that my train was on time, and I will see him tomorrow at 11 a.m. I spoke to a dear friend, where we laughed at our ridiculous slants on adult life, with no idea what we are doing, other than to hold hope.

As I scrolled through my Instagram and Facebook memories, I saw Emily and me smiling on the beach. So, I messaged her. On my Spotify playlist, a Bali chant blasted out, so I messaged my friend Lottie, too.

Today, while walking my highly sensitive and adorable Cavapoo, BoBo, I thought about a concept I recently read about: how there can be good love and bad love. But I don't believe bad love exists – the two words just don't belong in the same sentence. There is good love and then there is toxicity. We should never reason with toxic 'anything', especially when it comes to finding our happy home. Love does not torment, sick people do. Love does not want you to feel unsafe, abusers do. Love does not want you to negotiate with it. Love does not want you to forget its name. And love certainly does not want you to give up on love. I am now 43 years old and for the first time in my life, I'm so incredibly proud of the woman I am today. Some days I wobble, some days I can't see beyond the next hour, but I always trust in life, knowing that I've been here before – the heaviness, the loss, the lost loves – and look, I'm still here, talking to you. As long as our hearts are beating, healing and recovery have a chance.

And now, I'm a published author ... a PUBLISHED AUTHOR! I made it.

I am learning what it means to take the running shoes off and just be still. I don't fear change or crave rituals, because nothing ever stays the same. I get to love my people, daily. I am friends with women who continue to show me what it means to show up in life. I am exploring the toe-curling blend of sex and intimacy, soberly. I no longer apologise because of what my body can't do, but love what it can.

Gosh, just breathing is a gift.

As for the loves, they may come and they may go.

Some will disappear.

Some will orbit you, silently.

Some will remain friends, and help you with your end-of-year tax return.

Some will call a decade later and apologise.

Some will feature in an article with you, or a televised interview.

Some will buy a cat to avoid hard conversations (particularly when you're medically allergic to cats).

Some will stick, perfectly.

We can just never tell what will come of our 'loves'.

We can only do what is best for us.

Finding a love, be it friendship, family, romantic or otherwise, is as powerful as embryonic conception. The sheer number of moving parts that have to perfectly align at any given moment is like a universal orgasm. We need chemistry, timing, health, pleasure, openness, hope, and a 'slippery soul' to connect with the people who are meant for us.

Never question your worth.

Never deny yourself true happiness, and never take your eye off love.

Because love is a gift, and never a given.

TO THE WORLD THAT I AM TRULY GRATEFUL FOR

There are people who have loved me, saved me and inspired me. There are people who have picked me up in my breakdowns and meltdowns and encouraged me to ugly ... actually, beautifully cry.

On the days when my heart was broken, I would be helped out of bed. In the years when I didn't know another way, earth's wingless angels would make me some tea. On the days when I stood on a stage, the perfect encouraging nod was given.

Before I unravel into a gratitude-mess heap, I want to say thank you to ... you.

Thank you for holding this book between your hopeful hands. Thank you for trusting me with your curious mind. Thank you for staying with me through the moments that I am less than proud of. Thank you for believing that there is hope, there is happiness, and there is a different story to tell.

I haven't met you in person, but I feel like I have, or one day will. I hope you feel the same way too.

So, here goes.

My mummie, all these years you have encouraged me to speak my truth, without judgement from myself or others. You have made me feel so loved. You are braver and more humble than you'll ever know. I know we were meant to be paired up all those years ago. This is the kind of love that is hard to explain. But you get it. That moment our fingertips meet every morning, that is the love. I couldn't have written this book without you, because you guided me back home, time and time again.

Daddy, I love you. You are my solid ground. You are generous, honest, wise and gentle. You have supported me telling this story, despite it being hard for a father to hear. You have made me feel safe and free to be the person writing this today. Everyone needs a dad like you. I am the luckiest daughter there is.

My big brother, Andrew. I will always be your little sister, who will laugh at life with you. So, here we are, tag-teaming our Aussie adventures. You truly deserve love and happiness, always.

To Jan, you've been just the perfect second mum. I was just a teenager when we met, and honestly, I couldn't have wished for a more perfect step-mum. Thank you for always soothing my dating dilemmas; for sipping coffee on the Devonshire waterfront; for being such a beautiful friend. You love my dad, and in turn, you love me. I am so lucky that you've been such a huge and loving person in my life. Your quiet and humble generosity always makes such a HUGE impact. Blessed am I.

BoBo, our loving dog. BoBo, how unexpected but perfectly timed you were when you came into our lives. You're complex, and sensitive, and unpredictable, and funny, and lovable, and loyal, and noisy, and licky. I sometimes think that 'Esme' sent you to us; like a tiny piece of her lives in you. It's a joy to love you. We are your home, and you are ours.

Amy Molloy, gosh, where do I begin? I have never been more grateful for sweaty trainers and traumatic pasts. We always joked that you were six months ahead of me, because in many ways it was true. Sometimes, more than six months. Before I met you, I didn't know how to heal. I didn't have the faith in myself that I could. Not only have you edited my story, you rebuilt my heart. You have made me want to live a different way, with a different kind of love. Thank you.

Amy R, I will never forget the text message that cemented our friendship. When I was heartbroken, abandoned and grief-stricken, you sent me a picture of a spade. It was the digital symbol to say: I am here to dig you out of this pain. And you did. You have listened to me, encouraged me and nurtured me in ways only a best friend can. Your bravery is why women must never stop believing in their worth. You are a woman who is courageous, humble and insanely steeped in a constant desire for something bigger. My Bondi years felt safer, bolder and more brilliant, because you were my neighbour, my friend and my person. And you still are. I love you.

My sister mermaid, Chrissie, the ocean was our playground. Diving through a swell was easier with you. You taught me to clutch for the sand, and you taught me to clutch at love. In one of my most unforgettable classes, you asked, 'What would love do?' I have never forgotten this important reminder, and I have never forgotten our Bali adventure. Women like you remain forever grateful for and respectful of love. It doesn't come easy, and we are women who wouldn't want it to be. You are powerful, and you are loved. P.S. You never judged my Sunday hangovers and, in the Bondi yoga circuit, that was hard to suppress. So much love for you.

OMG, all this love is too perfect.

Jaqi, where would I be without you? We built a community from scratch, by being the creative, classic and original Aussie advocates that we are. You are one of the gentlest souls I know, and I can't imagine my life without you in it. May we one day rendition 'Hold On' by the band Wilson Phillips, with the same gusto we've always had for our friendship. Please say hello to my Aussie surrogate parents, 'Mama Carol and Papa Frank'.

Isla, you healed my heart ... plain and simple. We met because of our gorgeous friend, Imogen, and didn't that work out so wonderfully well? Every day, you teach me how to heal, recover, dream and accept life while we wait for more dreams to arrive. You are so brilliantly beautiful, inside and out. Wherever you are in the world, chasing breaking news and the next big story, I will happily wave you off – because I know there is always a voice note coming my way. Thank you for getting me here.

Mary, this is making me a little weepy to write, because, just today, you praised me for getting this book published, despite how terrifying it is. You have scoped my grammar and written the most perfect back-of-book blurb. As I write this, I know we're on to brilliant things in the creative and literary world. But more importantly, I will always remember the day, over a Diet Coke and plate of chips, you told me your story. It was then, as my eyes clogged up with tears, I knew we'd be friends. And now look at us, doing womanhood on our own terms. You, my friend, have changed my life. It's so scary bringing a book into the world, and you've been there, every single step of the way. I am sorry for asking you to plunge into the winter sea, but I am not sorry for how it made me admire our friendship even more.

I can't see through my glasses because of the tears. One sec, while I go wash them off and come back to you with a braver heart.

Sne, I will never forget the day you said, 'When I think of inviting a person into my life, I question, do I need them, or do I want them?' I have never forgotten this hearty formula. Thank you for being my Bondi family and welcoming me into your world. I will never forget reading your girls a bedtime story, and their faces when I told them how I relish Tim Tams for breakfast. You may be 10,000 miles away, but you are a woman who has changed, shaped and encouraged me to be the woman I am today. Love to you all.

Nikki P, well ... if there is a friendship that can successfully span an ocean, it's ours. Your humour, support, wit and persistence to want 'better' for us has been a driving force behind so many of my decisions. I love our bawdiness, random moments of creative genius and tender check-ins. Let's always keep bringing each other 'back to life'! I love you.

Nicky E, we met in the most random way and most special of spaces. But, if there is a woman who wears her heart on her sleeve, it's you. Our quarterly cocktail days, Victoria Beckham showdowns and plant-based catch-ups are some of the absolute highlights of my year. Thank you for showing me unconditional support and kindness. You are one of life's finest. I know Kylie will feel the same way about you too. Thank you for accepting my friend request, you gorgeous human, you.

Lissie, I can feel a little tear lurking at the back of my throat. If I had to visually create the love I have for you, it looks a little bit like candy floss: gentle, sweet, comforting. You are constantly reminding me how far our strength can take us. You make me feel safe in my scrappiest of moments. You have always been there for me, even when we were just starting out as friends. You are one of life's angels.

Sapna, had it not been for you, I'd never have been able to get out of Australia when I did. You helped me come 'home'. From a photoshoot to an Airbnb booking, to creative consulting, I've held you so close to the life that you helped me create. I think you're brilliant. You not only host my website, but you host our friendship, because without you, I wouldn't be back in Blighty! Let's hug soon, please.

Charlie, I remember the day when you invited me to join the MRKH Connect board, and, well, it was a day that felt like an MRKH homecoming. I admire your ethos, determination, loyalty, and the way you sign every message off with 'xxx' (I secretly love this!). You mean every word you say, and you do it with grace, loyalty and humour (even when strolling through the Houses of Parliament). If MRKH had to happen, then I am glad that it did – because it brought me to you.

Jennie G, how perfect that a 'viral vagina reel' connected us. You are my 'Jennie from LA', whom I boast about often, because you are one of the most talented, gifted and tenacious women I know. I remain so ridiculously thankful that you opened your doors to me when my heart felt closed. Thank you for welcoming me into your home, where I got to fall in love with you and the boys a little bit more. Thank you for re-opening my heart (and for taking me to that insane lesbian pool party!). Our type of friendship is the type that withstands geography and time. With gratitude, let me be your nurturer, forever.

Imogen, we've yet to embrace each other for our first squeeze, yet somehow, I feel like we've been friends forever. You have taught me how to usher in silence in the noise of trauma. You've shown me how to trust in the absolute unknown. You've taught me that connections are far more than a 'follow'. I adore being in your world and I consider myself oh, so lucky. P.S. Thank you for the introduction to Isla. This is the POWER of women coming together; a power I didn't know existed until I met you.

Michelle, 'Geez Louise'. I can't even try to compete with your infectious and comedic brain. But I do know that you guided me through the rockiness of change. If there was a definition of 'how to belly laugh at love, loss and life', the search would display 'Michelle Ahern: made in Australia'. If you ever find yourself eating soup in Spain alone, text me. Never stop being you ... NEVER, EVER STOP BEING YOU!

Ellamae, well, our little U-turn vaginas brought us together; our cul-de-sac anatomy made this friendship the perfection that it is. Sometimes, I run out of ways to say 'thank you'. But, Ellamae, thank you. You have created a world where taboo, stigma and silence serves no purpose, but shouting loudly about 'vaaaggggiiiinnnnnnnaaaaas' does. If we only ever catch up on podcasts, just tell me where to sign up for ours. I love you.

Nattie K, you are perfection. Whether you are flying above the sea saving lives in a helicopter, taking life-saving treatment to the streets of Sydney or rolling out your yoga mat next to mine, your loyalty to our friendship means the absolute world to me. You are the woman who reminds me daily, that a woman can be everything she chooses to be. I absolutely adore you.

Vics, you were and are so brave. It's been a privilege seeing your world unfurl into a happy, empowered and purposeful existence. Thank you for choosing me to hold your hand. I will never, ever let go. Keep shooting for stars!

Yogatime, the sandstone sanctuary that has witnessed my breakdowns, breakups and breakthroughs. The Balinese nook in Bondi, where I made some of my best decisions. I will never forget how, in this very one space, I was introduced to a life of acceptance, spirituality and wobbly headstands. I hope that everyone heals in this studio like I did. Wiebke, thank you, darling.

Jackie B, I remember the day I got home from therapy and said, 'I don't want to do this hard thing,' and you replied, 'We will do this hard thing together.' I mean, if that's not the most loyal friend, I don't know who is. You are beautiful, worthy, funny and perfect. Thank you for always lighting up my phone with, 'How are you and mama?' You are made of pure gold, and I am so pleased that we get to share this friendship together .

The 'Hensley' family: we are one solid family. We are a family that fights fit, with loyalty and dedication. We know our roots and remain proud of them. We know our collective worth. We know our immediate love. The 'Hensley' spirit is everything.

MRKH Connect, the brilliant UK flagship for people with MRKH, I am so honoured and privileged to be part of the team. Once upon a time, England was the landmark of my trauma, and now, it's the milestone for my purpose. I am so grateful for the invitation to come on board. We all do such brilliant work, and every week, we do something better. Every week we do something important. This book has happened because of the power behind the formidable MRKH community. Let's never stop believing in a better future for people with MRKH.

Ben W, you were the first phone call I made after leaving the London hospital. You were so kind, supportive and caring (I particularly loved you bringing me videos of *Jerry Springer* reruns!). As my then boyfriend, and now good friend, here we are, 26 years later, still supporting one another. What a special man you are. What a special friendship we have. Thank you.

Laura P, we make a formidable creative duo, and I am so grateful to you for being the talented *Stigma Shakers* podcast producer (and good friend!!). Your brain is brilliant and so are you. Thank you for coming into my life, because solo success can be a daunting place, and now, I don't have to celebrate alone.

Jenny Todd, my brilliant literary agent, you are just all shades of fabulous. Not only did you see my book as one worthy of exploring, but in turn, we talked about 'vaginas' for hours (erm, amazing!). Now, that's what I call the right fit between agent and author. The day I signed with you, alongside the twists and turns we've taken, was one of the best days of my life. Thank you for 'seeing' me.

My friends, Amy and Christina, the incredible women behind the Beautiful You MRKH Foundation, your invitation for me to write for you unleashed me from my shame. Thank you for trusting my words, and for trusting me. The world will always be a better place, because your conviction and courage said so. I will never forget you both.

Oh, the adorable Dr Susan Carroll, I wouldn't change a thing about my past, because without that pain, I wouldn't have met you. You are gentle, wise and brilliant. I know you will go down in history as being one of the all-time greats for people like us. Had it not been for you, I would have boarded a flight out of Chicago, when my nerves were 100 per cent frayed. You supported me then, and you continue to support me now. Friend, I love you.

This wouldn't be a story without mentioning the first person to openly talk about MRKH ... ever! Esther Leidolf, you took the historical brunt for us, to make our 'now' better. Thank you for digging deep into your courage and for telling your story with such passion. Meeting you was like meeting a celebrity. Now, you are my dear celebrity friend. I will do everything to make sure the world always knows about Esther's courage.

Without you, the MRKH community, I wouldn't have found my other family. You are one of the fiercest groups of powerhouse survivors I have ever come across. Perhaps none of us wanted this life, but I do know that this diagnosis has given me friendships for life. Keep going – you've got this!

To all those behind my broken hearts, I know that we were in pain. I am not angry. I am grateful. You helped me find peace, and in turn, I hope you did too. Wherever you are, be happy, ex-boyfriends.

To the cutesy British country pub, The Cross Keys, Pangbourne, I will always be super grateful for my writing nook. Yours truly, 'Little Miss Thursday'.

You were never a pet, Dolly, you were my best friend. The cutest, quirkiest Chihuahua there ever was. Thank you for exposing me to a love that is only made for mothers. I love you exactly this way.

I know, Esme, that somewhere you are loving me and I am loving you back. Keep reminding me, in your way, that you are still close to me. And thank you for choosing me.

And again, to you, my reader.

You are LOVE.

Keep going, keep living, keep hoping.

Go gently.

Ally xo

Printed in Dunstable, United Kingdom

64784422R00119